Compl Dropping Acid Reflux Diet Cookbook.

Easy Anti Acid Diet Meal Plans & Recipes to Heal GERD and LPR

This document is geared towards providing exact and reliable information in regards to the topic and issue covered. The publication is sold with the idea that the publisher is not required to render an accounting, officially permitted, or otherwise, qualified services. If advice is necessary, legal or professional, a practiced individual in the profession should be ordered.

From a Declaration of Principles which was accepted and approved equally by a Committee of the American Bar Association and a Committee of Publishers and Associations.

The information herein is offered for informational purposes solely and is universal as so. The presentation of the information is without a contract or any type of guarantee assurance.

The trademarks that are used are without any consent, and the publication of the trademark is without permission or backing by the trademark owner. All trademarks and brands within this book are for clarifying purposes only and are owned by the owners themselves, not affiliated with this document.

Table of Contents

Introduction

Numerous health conditions can be effectively treated and reversed with dietary and lifestyle changes. Gastrointestinal reflux disease or GERD is one such health complexity-common among many patients yet one of the least understood. Acidic reflux is neither ordinary nor temporary, as many people falsely suspect that it diminishes with time; rather, our efforts can proactively alleviate the progression of the problem. According to American Society for Gastrointestinal Endoscopy, acid reflux is defined in these words: *"Gastroesophageal reflux is a chronic disease that occurs when stomach contents flow back (reflux) into the food pipe (esophagus). It is usually caused by failure of the muscle valve (called the lower esophageal sphincter) between the stomach and the esophagus to close properly. The backwash of stomach acid irritates the lining of the lower esophagus and causes the symptom of heartburn."*

In brief, the acid reflux diet properly restricts the consumption of acid forming foods, including high fats, excessive carbs, and complex protein cuisines. Such food can increase the production of HCl in the stomach, so much that it splashes back into the esophagus and damages the inner lining of the track. It further causes a tightening of the LES, lower esophageal sphincter, leading to regurgitation and heartburning. Through this book, a possible course of action to prevent and treat Acid reflux is delivered, while identifying the major causes and common symptoms. With clear understanding, anyone suffering from GERD can curb the problem.

Part-1

Chapter-1. Understanding Acid Reflux and GERD:

Acid Alkaline Balance for good Health and Diet:

Acid reflux is a common health problem experienced by all, irrespective of the genetics, age and size of the person. According to a 2014 survey, about 30 percent of the US population is suffering from GERD and this percent included people from different genders, all ages and body sizes. It becomes a routine for many sufferers, since most individuals are unfamiliar with the effectiveness of treatment through a dietary plan. Conversely, most people seek medications, which prove harmful in the longer run. The main crux of the acid reflux diet is to allow a better acid-alkaline balance in the diet for better health. Acid reflux is a state when a person feels one's heart burning or burning sensations in the stomach ("Gastroesophageal Reflux (GER) and Gastroesophageal Reflux Disease (GERD) in Adults, 2014). Highly strong HCl is produced in the stomach to digest proteins initially. When more acidic food is eaten, it aggravates the acidic condition and causes reflux, which is readily sensed by the upper sphincter of the stomach and lower esophageal walls; as a result, a sensation of burning is produced. Acidic food can be described as any edible which can stimulate the stomach to produce more acid- (*National Institute of Food Agriculture (USDA-NIFA)*). Other than food, there are several underlying causes of acid reflux.

What causes acid reflux?

Here are some of the commonly known causes of acid reflux, which can either exacerbate the condition or aggravate it.

1. Gut problems:

A hiatal hernia is a typical cause for acid reflux. It occurs due to the movement of the lower esophageal sphincter LES and upper stomach portion over the diaphragm. In turn, the acid reaches the esophagus.

2. Pregnancy:

It is quite common in all the pregnant women, especially during the first pregnancy. It resonates from hormonal imbalances, which are natural and can be controlled with medications.

3. Smoking:

Acid reflux is common in smokers, and it occurs when the esophageal walls are damages due to constant smoking. The smoke also leads to more acid secretion, loss of muscle function, less saliva production, damaged mucous membranes and decreased reflexes.

4. Diet:

Unhealthy diet is the primary reason for acid reflux. There are certain food items that expedite heartburning and acid reflux, including alcohol, spicy food, drinks, chocolate, fatty meals, etc.

Additional reasons that perpetuate acid reflux further reflect obesity, sleeplessness, large meals, and heavy medicines.

Symptoms of Acid Reflux:

It is a popular myth that heartburning or discomfort in the stomach is the only symptom of acid reflux, which is far from true. Heartburn is symptom major sign of acid refluxes and a serious one. Yet many other symptoms also indicate acid reflux at some level:

1. As stated above, heartburn is one of the obvious acid reflux signs. It is felt because of the acidic damage to the lower end of the esophagus; it is a passage that connects the mouth with the stomach. Due to the reflux acid reaching the esophagus, it produces a feeling of intense burning.

2. Regurgitation: Based on acid reflux, a person feels a constant expulsion of undigested food from the stomach into the esophagus, which sometimes crosses the pharynx.

3. Bloating: bloating is the direct outcome of acidity in the stomach. While it is a not primary symptom of acid reflux, it can be deemed as a sign.

4. Bloody or black stools or bloody vomiting: when food is not digested properly or intense acidity damages the internal lining of the gut, these failures may result in such a condition. Consult a doctor immediately.

5. Burping: the huge volume of gas is produced in the stomach when there is excess acid to digest the food. It reacts by producing gas, which causes unwanted or constant burping.

6. Dysphagia: Again, this serious symptom happens when the esophagus starts to narrow down, and it feels like food is stuck in the throat. It makes it difficult to swallow food.

7. Nausea: that heaviness and acidity in the stomach cause nausea.

8. Weight loss for no known reason: sudden weight loss is never a good sign. A person with acid reflux can also experience weight loss.

9. In extreme cases, acid reflux can also result in wheezing, dry cough, hoarseness, or a chronic sore throat.

Dietary Acid Damage: Why It should be feared?

An acidic diet can be harmful to people with chronic kidney conditions, since they are more prone to a higher risk of kidney failure when they ingest acidic foods. They are therefore prescribed to eat more fruits and vegetables while reducing the amount of high fat and meat in the meal. Acid damage should always be feared, even at the earliest stage; the progressive damage can lead to bigger health problems. It severely impairs the stomach walls, its secretary glands, and walls of the esophagus.

Acid Reflex, Esophagus, and Cancer:

In acid reflux, the acid from the stomach splashes back into the lower part of the esophagus. The stomach is designed in such a way that its internal walls can bear the low pH of the HCl, but the inner lining of the esophagus cannot. It does not have protective tissues or cells to defend against the acid, which is why acid reflux always inflicts damage in the inner layer of the esophagus.

Such damage can lead to a special condition known as Barrett's esophagus; the term was first coined by Australian thoracic surgeon Norman Barrett in 1950. It is the body's natural response to replace the inner cells with tissues similar to the tissues in the intestinal area. The process of replacement can often provoke the development of precancerous cells. Even though people with Barrett's esophagus are highly susceptible to cancer, the majority rarely develop esophageal cancer. Yet people with acid reflux and Barrett's condition are more prone to esophageal cancer than others. They are twice the times more susceptible to cancer, as the WebMD survey suggests.

The esophagus links the mouth with the stomach, and the passage is neutral to an alkaline atmosphere. However, any problem in the stomach can damage the lower the part of the passage. Constant acid reflux can cause cancer in the esophageal cells, and itt can be spread easily into the entire body through the digestive system. It can act as an epicenter of cancer. According to the Cancer Treamtent Centers of America, there are two types of cancer that can occur in the esophagus: carcinoma and adenocarcinoma. Cancer patients, therefore, are prescribed an anti acid diet.

To further protect the esophagus from cancer, it is important to guard it from Barrett's condition and most importantly from the acid reflux. There are few simple rules to deal with the problem at hand. First, shed the risks associated with obesity and lose some weight if you are overweight. Then avoid lying down right after eating. It can cause a splash of acid into the esophagus. While sleeping, the head and chest should be positioned in such a way that they remain above the level of the stomach. Whenever a person experiences acidity or reflux, he should try taking some antacids to counter the effects. Smoking and drinking should be avoided to reduce the risks of acid reflux and esophageal cancer. Adding more fruits and vegetables to one's diet is also advised.

Acid Reflux and Weight Gain:

Any digestive disorder can lead to obesity and weight gain. But why is this correlation true? That is what happens when food is not digested properly and not absorbed into the required proportions. There are several studies to validate this claim. Gastroesophageal reflux disease GERD is connected to obesity as per the claims of *Jacobson, 2006*.

Effects of Acid Alkaline Imbalance:

Acid-alkaline imbalance in the diet is quite crucial in maintaining the internal climate of the body. Each part of the gut has an atmosphere of its own, and a diet disrupting this balance can cause medical complications such as indigestion, esophageal cancer, obesity, etc. According to 2006 book, *The Great Physician's Rx for Heartburn and Acid Reflux,* Rubin &Brasco attribute the root cause of all the diseases relating to autotoxication occurs because of acidic accumulation. Ever since then, a balanced acid alkaline diet has been used to treat and prevent all such diseases. It prescribes the intake of a less acidic and a more alkaline diet.

Testing for pH Balance:

There are several different methods to test the pH balance within the body. It can be measure through saliva, urine, and blood. All three tests can be carried out separately using the pH testing strips. Each strip is dipped in the given sample and left until color appears. Next that color is matched with the scales given on the box to identify the pH values of the sample.

Chapter 2. Relationship Between Food & Symptoms.

Understanding the Role of protein, Carbohydrates, and Fats in Healing

Dietary Acid Damage:

The acid produced excessively in the stomach due to the high protein, high fats, and high carb food can damage the internal cells of the stomach and esophagus. The role of every macronutrient cannot be denied, but they all have to be taken in suitable proportions and in a required amount by the body. Lean proteins, low carbs, and low fats should be targeted to minimize the acid reflux and the damage.

Acidity and Alkalinity:

When you examine a pH scale, it marks everything as acidic if the substance has a pH value lower than 7, whereas values higher than 7 indicate alkalinity. This same rule is applied to the food, our blood, saliva, and the internal gut. The saliva and blood are both slightly alkaline in nature, to maintain this value, only an alkaline diet can yield effective results.

There is a term, most commonly used to define the acid-alkaline balance in the food, called Dietary Acid Load (DAL): the greater the dietary acid load, the more the food becomes unsuitable for the acid reflux diet, (*Division of Nephrology and Hypertension, Department of Medicine, University of*

Miami Miller School of Medicine, Miami, FL, USA). The load is actually determined by a calculation of the ratios of acid-inducing foods and the alkaline forming foods in the meal. Animal proteins are generally acid at the end forming, as they contain methionine, which produces sulfuric acid when digested- *(Finkelstein, 1990).* The acid effects can be neutralized by partaking in more fruits and vegetables.

In the prehistoric days, the human diet was more dependent on the plant sources, which were more alkaline in nature. Therefore, the whole human body, including the kidneys and the guts, evolved to function more on an alkaline diet. Contrary to that, the human diet today is shifting more towards the animal sources and acid forming food source. This alteration in the diet results in the number of health problems, including acid reflux. According to a 2014 report by for *the Centers for Disease Control and Prevention Chronic Kidney Disease Surveillance Team*, about 12000 Americans were found at the increased risks of kidney damage due to the greater dietary acid load.

Breaking Acid-Generation Habits and Establishing Acid-Reduction Practices:

We are the generation of poor eating habits, and this routine has to break in order to avoid severe problems like acid reflux.

1. All vegetables, especially the green leafy ones, are healthy for people suffering from acid reflux. Avocados, spinach, kale, and lettuce are far better than eating heavy meats and grains.
2. Reducing the amount of acidic food intake can also decrease the chances of GERD. Such food includes sugar, dairy, and red meat, etc.
3. Alcohol disrupts the entire digestive functioning, and it is extremely acidic in nature. In sum, it must be avoided at most.
4. Drinking alkaline water can also help, and it gives instant relief to the stomach. It keeps the acid-alkaline balance in the body.
5. Energy boosting drinks are so rich in sugar that they instantly produce more acid. Such drinks should be replaced with the natural juices and nectars.
6. Routine exercise can keep the metabolism working and reduce the chances of the acidity. 30 minutes of exercise in a day is vital to control GERD.
7. Stress and emotional turmoil can also disrupt the sync of the digestive hormones, resulting in acid reflux. In brief, it should be avoided through meditation and therapies.

Food Allergies, Sensitivities and Intolerance:

Different people react to different food differently. Some people are more intolerant towards carbohydrates, whereas others may experience allergies due to protein. Acid reflux can also be the typical result of such allergies. In such cases, a person should recognize the food causing the reflux and the allergies. After understanding the intolerance, only then it can be treated. According to the *Division of Asthma, Allergy and Lung Biology, Department of Paediatric Allergy, King's College London, Guy's and St. Thomas' Hospitals NHS Foundation Trust, London, UK, the* following are the five main symptoms of food intolerance:

- Eczema, skin rashes, hives, etc.
- Asthma, running nose, nose, and ear infections
- Depression, anxiety, restlessness, etc.
- Headaches or migraines
- Mouth ulcers, stomach aches, constipation, urinary urgency, diarrhea, etc.

Avoid Acid Reflux By Specific Diets

Acid reflux can only be treated by making certain changes in the dietary routine. Other health-oriented diet plans cannot serve the purpose of avoiding the dangers of acid reflux. However, an alkaline can reduce the problem to an extent. A low fat, low carb, and clean protein diet is the answer to this problem in particular and any specific diet with such traits can serve the cause.

The Fiber Gap! How to Bridge it?

Fibers are important, whether you are following any dietary plan or not. For acid reduction, a fibrous diet is essential, and the intake can be enhanced by eating more fruits and leafy green vegetables. Increasing the organic items in a meal can enrich its fibers. In contrast, overcooked and processed meals deplete all fibers. Therefore, they all should be avoided and replaced with more fresh and organic food.

Developing Your pH Savvy: The Truth About Acid/Alkaline Balance and "Healthy" Foods, People with Acid Reflux Avoid

The first step is to achieve a clear understanding of the pH scale and different values of the food that you eat. By making a habit of reading the labels and by keeping a track record of daily meals, a person can avoid the burn of acid. Certain meals which are inappropriate for people with acid reflux include:

1. Dairy products
2. High-fat edibles
3. Sugars
4. Sugary drinks
5. High-fat meats

Chapter-3. Creating Acid-Alkaline Balance

It is not always easy to create a perfect acid-alkaline balance when you have to deal with the daily meal preparations. Planning and a clear understanding of the dietary targets and goals should be kept in mind. For GERD, such targets include:

1. Avoid Foods or Substances That Weaken Your LES:
Any food item that can weaken the lower esophageal sphincter (LES) has to be avoided- *American Society for Gastrointestinal Endoscopy.* High sugar substances, acidic forming food, and smoke from the cigarettes can all damage the LES, so these items should be restricted

2. Avoid Foods or Substances That Increase Acidity:
Saturated fats, processed flour, grains, and red meat proteins are acid forming substances should be omitted within an acid reflux diet.

3. Eat More Alkaline Foods:
Fruits and vegetables which are alkaline in nature are best to counter the acidity in the stomach, so there should be more alkaline foods in the diet than the acidic ones

4. Avoid Foods That May Increase IAP:

IAP is the autoimmune protocol (first coined by Dr. Loren Cordain) and is important to choose foods which can strengthen this system while rendering the body more tolerant towards any imbalance or strong against the diseases.

5. Eat Small Meals:

Small meals mean fewer burdens on the stomach and decreased production of the HCl, which results in lesser acidity. That is why eating small meals to avoid acidity is always suggested.

6. Stop Eating at Least Four Hours Before Bedtime:

Around bedtime, our metabolic process slows down, and the body cannot digest actively in the stomach. That is why it is advised to stop the eating at least 4 hours before going to sleep.

7. Wear Loose Clothing:

Loose clothing is important for those who are allergic and reactive to any sort of unease. Loose clothing relaxes the body and promotes healthy digestion.

8. If You are overweight, lose weight:

Obesity is strongly linked to acid reflux, so a person should lose weight to gain high metabolic rates in order to digest well without excessive acid formation.

9. Minimize Fat in Foods:

Fats are not easily digested. Therefore, excessive acid is produced in the gut to counter the incoming fatty food. To rectify, reduce all items which contain a high amount of saturated fats.

10.   Watch What (and When) You Drink:

Drinking can either relieve the condition or make it worse. Therefore, always look into the drinks' ingredients and avoid those containing high sugar, fats, or alcohol.

11.   Emergency Help for Flare-Ups:

Acid reflux should be taken seriously. At times it can be a symptom of heart issues or other fatal conditions. Call for emergency help when you feel intense burning in the stomach or in the chest.

Chapter-4. Food Tables

Foods Not to Eat

Acidic food manufactures more acidity, which is why patients suffering from GERD should avoid all such items. There are certain foods which can aggravate the acid reflux condition, and these types should be avoided and replaced with suitable alternatives. Sugar, for instance, can cause acidity in the stomach, so it can be substituted with other natural or low carb sweeteners.

The following foods worsen GERD and tend to be acidic in nature. Their intake should be lowered and reduced drastically.

• Foods with high fats and oils (these foods may result in relaxation of the sphincter in the stomach)

• Meats (if highly acidic in nature while having a higher amount of fatty acids and cholesterol levels)

• Food sources of saturated fats include cheese (highly acidic in nature) and milk.

• Excessive amounts of salts

• Mint

• Chocolate

• Carbonated beverages (sodas)

• Alcoholic drinks

• Caffeine

• Acidic drinks, which include coffee and orange juice etc.

• Acidic foods which consist of tomato sauce etc.

Foods to Eat

Following the acid reflux demands a certain restriction, but most of the delicious and healthy ingredients can still be enjoyed in the perfect combination. Unlike other health-oriented regimens, an acid reflux diet is a little less restrictive and allows more convenience. As long as you are not eating the acid forming foods, it is safe to enjoy anything. The list indicates permitted items below on an acid reflux diet:

Fruits	Vegetabl es	Meat Beans	Dairy	Grains	Fats and nuts
Apple	Potato	Lean Beef	Cheese	Bread	Almonds
Banana	Broccoli	Egg whites	Cream cheese, fat-free	Cereal	Brazil nuts
Melons	Cabbage	Chicken	Sour cream, fat-free	Cornbread	Chestnut s
Avocados	Carrots	Tofu	Soy cheese, low fat	Pretzel	Pumpkin seeds
Mango	Green beans	Beans		Brown rice	Sesame seeds

Peaches	Peas	Fish		White rice	Flaxseeds
strawberries	Zucchini	Shrimp		Rice cakes	Sunflowe r seeds
Papayas	Artichokes	Mussels		Graham crackers	
Pears		Prawns			
Raisins		Lamb			

BREAKFAST AND BRUNCH RECIPES

Spiced Apricot Oats

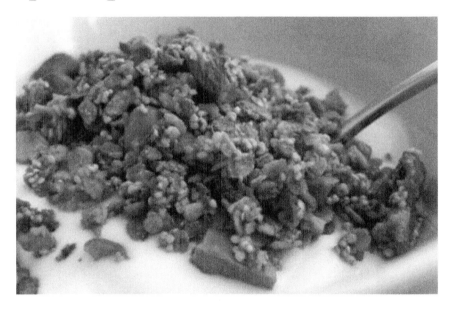

Ingredients:

- 2 cups whole rolled oats

- 1/2 cups soft dried apricots, chopped

- 1/3 cup soft dried figs, chopped

- 1/4 cup soft pitted dates, chopped

- 1/4 cup dried apple slices, chopped

- 1/6 cup dried coconut

- 1 teaspoon ground ginger

- 2 teaspoon mixed spice

- 5 egg whites

How to prepare:

1. Set the oven to 150 degrees C.

2. Layer a baking sheet with parchment paper.

3. Mix everything in a bowl except egg whites.

4. Stir in egg whites and mix again.

5. Spread the mixture in the baking tray.

6. Bake for 40 mins approximately.

7. Slice and serve.

Preparation time: 15 minutes

Cooking time: 40 minutes

Total time: 55 minutes

Servings: 4

Nutritional Values:

- *Calories 519*
- *Total Fat 31.4 g*
- *Saturated Fat 25.9 g*
- *Cholesterol 0 mg*
- *Sodium 99 mg*
- *Total Carbs 57.8 g*
- *Fiber 8.7 g*
- *Sugar 2.3 g*
- *Protein 6.5 g*

Banana and Blackberry Smoothie Bowl

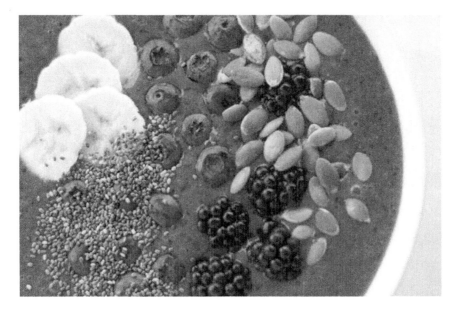

Ingredients:

- 2 teaspoon pumpkin seeds

- 2 teaspoon sunflower seeds

- 2 small bananas, frozen

- 11/4 cup blackberries

- 1/3 cup 0% fat Greek-style yogurt

- 1/4 cup apple juice

- 1 teaspoon porridge oats

- 2 tablespoons lemon juice (optional)

- 2 small ripe figs, sliced

How to prepare:

1. Toast all the seeds in a skillet over medium heat for
    minutes.

2. Blend bananas with yogurt and blackberries in a blender.

3. Pour the smoothies in the serving bowl and top with figs, blackberries, and toasted seeds.

Preparation time: 5 minutes

Cooking time: 01 minutes

Total time: 6 minutes

Servings: 2

Nutritional Values:

- *Calories 544*
- *Total Fat 24.9 g*
- *Saturated Fat 4.7 g*
- *Cholesterol 194 mg*
- *Sodium 607 mg*
- *Total Carbs 30.7 g*
- *Fiber 1.4 g*
- *Sugar 3.3 g*
- *Protein 6.4g*

Banana breakfast loaf

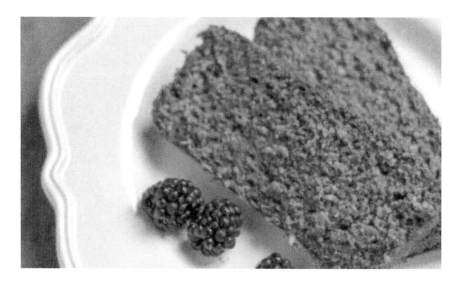

Ingredients:

- 4 large bananas
- 2 egg whites
- 1/2 cups dates, finely chopped
- 3 heaped tablespoon low-fat Greek-style yogurt
- 1/4 cup dried coconut
- 2 tablespoon chia seeds
- 2 ¼ cup almond flour
- ¼ teaspoon bicarbonate of soda
- 1 teaspoon mixed spice
- 2-3 tablespoon almond milk

How to prepare:

1. Set the oven to 320 degrees F. Line a loaf pan with parchment.

2. Mash 3 bananas with a whisk in egg whites.

3. Stir in coconut, chia seeds, dates, and yogurt.

4. Mix flour with soda and spices. Add this mixture to the yogurt mixture.

5. Stir in 2 tablespoons and mix until smooth.

6. Pour the batter into the loaf tin.

7. Top the batter with sliced bananas. Bake for 30 minutes.

8. Slice and serve.

Preparation time: 10 minutes

Cooking time: 30 minutes

Total time: 40 minutes

Servings: 4

Nutritional Values:

- *Calories 408*
- *Total Fat 16.5 g*
- *Saturated Fat 5 g*
- *Cholesterol 8 mg*
- *Sodium 285 mg*
- *Total Carbs 56.1 g*
- *Fiber 8.7 g*
- *Sugar 10.1 g*
- *Protein 11 g*

Plum and almond porridge

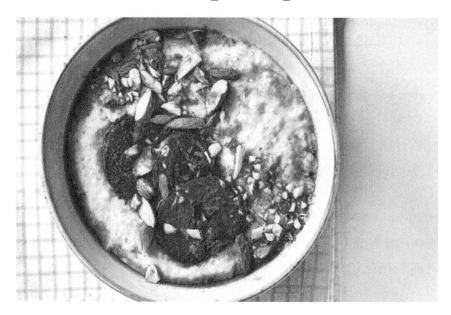

Ingredients:

- 6 small plums, halved and stoned
- 2 tablespoon maple syrup, plus extra to serve
- ¼ teaspoon ground cinnamon
- 1 orange, zested and juiced
- 1/2 cups porridge oats
- 1/4 cup oat bran
- 1/4 cup quinoa
- 1 ½ cup unsweetened almond milk
- 2 tablespoon almonds, roughly chopped

How to prepare:

1. Set the oven to 320 degrees F. Spread the plums in a baking
2. Add cinnamon and maple syrup on top.

3. Toss the plum and bake them for 25 minutes.
4. Drizzle orange juice on top and bake for another 5 minutes.
5. Cook porridge oats with quinoa, oat bran, water, and almond milk in a cooking pot for 20 minutes.
6. Serve the porridge with the 3 plums mixture, almond, and orange zest.

Preparation time: 10 minutes
Cooking time: 30 minutes
Total time: 40 minutes
Servings: 2

Nutritional Values:

- *Calories 284*
- *Total Fat 7.9 g*
- *Saturated Fat 0 g*
- *Cholesterol 36 mg*
- *Sodium 704 mg*
- *Total Carbs 46 g*
- *Fiber 3.6 g*
- *Sugar 5.5 g*
- *Protein 7.9 g*

Bircher muesli

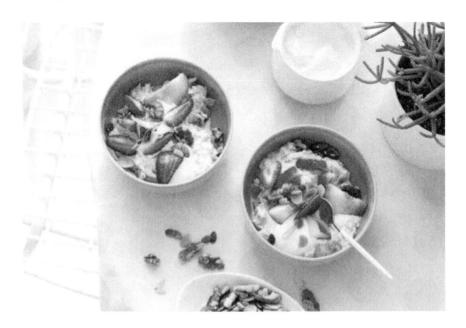

Ingredients:

- 2 1/4 cup oats
- 1/4 cup (2oz) raisins
- 1/4 cup dried apricots, chopped
- 1/4 cup (2½oz) flaked almonds
- 2 eating Rosedene Farms apples
- 2 cups almond milk
- 1/2 cup orange juice
- juice of ½ Suntrail Farms lemon
- 11/4 cup natural yogurt
- fresh berries, to serve

Method:

1. Mix oats with apricots, grated apples, almonds, and raisins in a bowl.

2. Stir in milk, lemon juice, and orange.

3. Mix well and refrigerate overnight.

4. Garnish with a dollop of yogurt.

5. Serve.

Preparation Time: 5 minutes

Cooking Time: 0 minutes

Total Time: 5 minutes

Servings: 2

Nutritional Values:

- *Calories 462*
- *Total Fat 1.5 g*
- *Saturated Fat 0.5 g*
- *Cholesterol 0 mg*
- *Total Carbs 119.8 g*
- *Dietary Fiber 10 g*
- *Sugar 78 g*
- *Protein 4.5 g*

Banana and Mango Smoothie

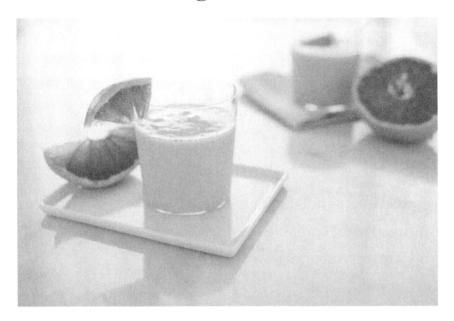

Ingredients:
- 1 small pink grapefruit, peeled and segmented
- 1 banana, peeled and chopped
- 1 mango, halved, stoned and flesh chopped
- 2 cups natural yogurt
- handful ice cubes

How to prepare:
1. Blend mango, grapefruit, and banana in a blender, along with yogurt and ice cubes.
2. Serve.

Preparation time: 10 minutes
Cooking time: 0 minutes

Total time: 10 minutes

Servings: 1

Nutritional Values:

- *Calories 134*
- *Total Fat 4.7 g*
- *Saturated Fat 0.6 g*
- *Cholesterol 0 mg*
- *Sodium 1 mg*
- *Total Carbs 54.1 g*
- *Fiber 7 g*
- *Sugar 23.3 g*
- *Protein 6.2 g*

Moroccan fritters

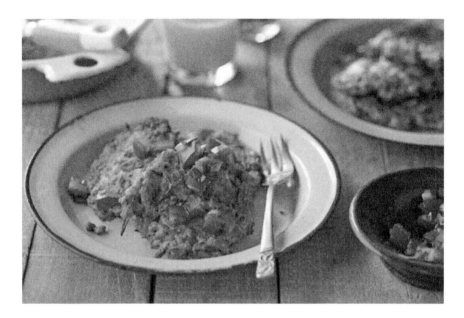

Ingredients:

- 1/3 cup almond flour
- 1 teaspoon baking powder
- 2 teaspoon ground cumin
- 2 teaspoon ground coriander
- 2 teaspoon dried mint
- 1/2 teaspoon salt
- 2 zucchinis, coarsely grated
- 4 spring onions, finely chopped
- olive oil, for frying

For the chili-pepper relish

- 2 red bell pepper, seeded and diced
- 1 large handful of chopped coriander leaves
- 1 medium-sized red chilli, seeded and diced
- juice of 1 lime

Method:

1. Combine baking powder with flour, spices, salt, and mint in a bowl.
2. Squeeze excess water from the zucchini using a paper towel.
3. Add these courgettes to the flour along with pepper and spring onions.
4. Stir in ¼ pint water and mix well. Let it sit for 10 minutes.
5. Meanwhile, mix all the ingredients for the relish in a small bowl.
6. Grease a nonstick skillet with cooking oil and preheat it over medium heat.
7. Pour ¼ of the batter into the skillet and cook for 2 minutes per side.
8. Keep the fritters on paper towels and serve with the relish.

Preparation Time: 10 minutes
Cooking Time: 15 minutes

Total Time: 25 minutes

Servings: 4

Nutritional Values:

- *Calories 387*
- *Total Fat 6 g*
- *Saturated Fat 9.9 g*
- *Cholesterol 41 mg*
- *Sodium 154 mg*
- *Total Carbs 37.4 g*
- *Fiber 2.9 g*
- *Sugar 15.3 g*
- *Protein 6.6 g*

Pancakes with Avocado

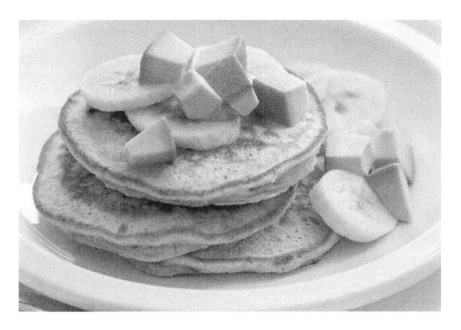

Ingredients:

- 2 small avocados
- 1 lime, juiced, plus extra halves, to serve
- handful chopped coriander

For the pancakes

- 1/3 cup (3oz) almond flour
- 2 egg whites
- ½ cup chicken stock
- 1 tablespoon Worcestershire or coconut aminos
- 1/4 cup (2oz) greens, shredded
- 1 carrot, grated
- 1 leek, trimmed and shredded
- 1 courgette, trimmed and grated

- 2 tablespoon sunflower oil

Method:

1. Mix flour with egg, Worcestershire sauce and stock in a large bowl.
2. Add vegetables to the batter and mix gently.
3. Grease a frying pan with cooking and preheat for 30 seconds.
4. Pour half of the batter into the pan and cook for 3 minutes per side.
5. Use remaining batter to cook more pancakes.
6. Mash avocado with seasoning and lime juice.
7. Serve the pancakes with avocado mash.

Preparation Time: 10 minutes
Cooking Time: 15 minutes
Total Time: 25 minutes
Servings: 4

Nutritional Value:
- *Calories 212*
- *Total Fat 11.8 g*
- *Saturated Fat 2.2 g*
- *Cholesterol 0 mg*
- *Sodium 321 mg*
- *Total Carbs 14.6 g*
- *Dietary Fiber 4.4 g*
- *Sugar 8 g*
- *Protein 17.3 g*

Dutch pancakes

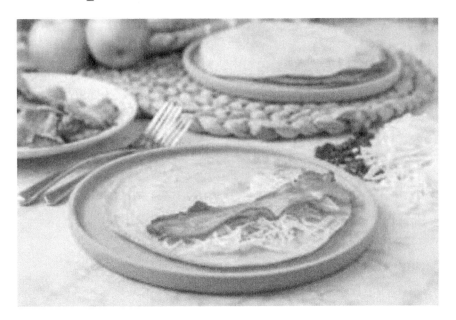

Ingredients:

- 21/4 cup almond flour
- 2 cups almond milk
- 2 egg whites
- pinch salt
- 2 tablespoons vegetable oil
- small bunch spring onions, chopped
- 3 sausages, torn into small pieces
- 1 (7oz) tin sweetcorn
- green salad, to serve

Method:

1. Combine egg whites with flour, salt, and milk in a mixing bowl and whisk until become creamy.
2. Heat butter in an ovenproof skillet on medium heat.
3. Divide the spring onions into four portions and sauté one portion until golden brown.
4. Pour in 1/4th of the batter and spread it into a thin layer.
5. Cook the pancake for 2 mins per side until golden brown.
6. Make more pancakes by repeating the same steps.
7. Serve warm with desired garnish.

Preparation Time: 15 minutes
Cooking Time: 15 minutes
Total Time: 30 minutes
Servings: 4

Nutritional Value:

- *Calories 412*
- *Total Fat 24.8 g*
- *Saturated Fat 12.4 g*
- *Cholesterol 3 mg*
- *Sodium 132 mg*
- *Total Carbs 43.8 g*
- *Dietary Fiber 13.9 g*
- *Sugar 21.5 g*
- *Protein 18.9 g*

French Crêpes with Bananas

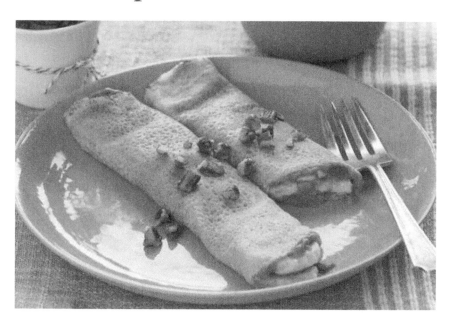

Ingredients:

- ½ cup almond flour
- ½ teaspoon gluten-free baking powder
- 2 medium egg whites, beaten
- 2 cups almond milk (or soy or rice milk)
- 5 teaspoon sunflower oil
- 4 bananas, peeled and sliced
- 2 teaspoon maple syrup (or honey)
- ¼ teaspoon ground cinnamon, plus extra to dust
- dairy-free yogurt, to serve
- 2 teaspoon pumpkin seeds, to garnish

How to prepare:

1. Whisk flour, salt, and baking powder in a mixing bowl.

2. Stir in milk and egg whites while whisking slowly until smooth.
3. Preheat sunflower oil in a nonstick skillet and add a ladle of batter.
4. Spread the batter into a pancake and cook for 2 minutes per side.
5. Make more pancakes and spread them onto the serving plate.
6. Add banana slices on top of each pancake and wrap them gently.
7. Serve.

Preparation time: 10 minutes
Cooking time: 15 minutes
Total time: 25 minutes
Servings: 04

Nutritional Values:

- *Calories 331*
- *Total Fat 2.5 g*
- *Saturated Fat 0.5 g*
- *Cholesterol 0 mg*
- *Sodium 595 mg*
- *Total Carbs 69 g*
- *Fiber 12.2 g*
- *Sugar 12.5 g*
- *Protein 8.7g*

APPETIZERS AND SIDES RECIPES

Playgroup Granola Bars

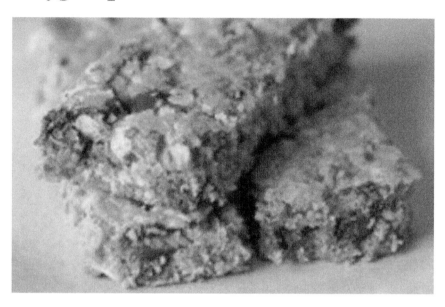

Ingredients:

- 2 cups rolled oats
- 3/4 cup packed coconut sugar
- 1/2 cup wheat germ
- 3/4 teaspoon ground cinnamon
- 1 cup almond flour
- 3/4 cup raisins (optional)
- 3/4 teaspoon salt
- 1/2 cup honey
- 1 egg, beaten
- 1/2 cup vegetable oil
- 2 teaspoons vanilla extract

How to prepare:

1. Set the oven at 350 degrees F to preheat. Grease a 9x13 inch pan with cooking spray.
2. Toss oats with wheat germ, flour, raisins, salt, cinnamon, and coconut sugar in a bowl
3. Add egg white, oil, vanilla, and honey to the mixture.
4. Mix well with your hands and then transfer it to the baking pan.
5. Bake for 35 mins until golden brown around the edges.
6. Slice and serve.

Preparation time: 10 minutes
Cooking time: 35 minutes
Total time: 45 minutes
Servings: 04

Nutritional Values:

- *Calories 307*
- *Total Fat 25 g*
- *Saturated Fat 5 g*
- *Cholesterol 16 mg*
- *Sodium 372 mg*
- *Total Carbs 16 g*
- *Fiber 5 g*
- *Sugar 4 g*
- *Protein 10 g*

Cocktail Meatballs

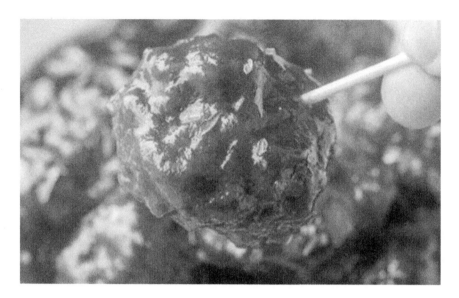

Ingredients:

- 1 pound lean ground beef
- 1 egg
- 4 tablespoons water
- 1/2 cup bread crumbs
- 3 tablespoons minced onion
- 1 (8 ounces) can jellied cranberry sauce
- 1/4 cup chili sauce
- 1 tablespoon coconut sugar
- ¼ cup apple cider vinegar

How to prepare:

1. Set the oven to 350 degrees F.
2. Combine beef with all other ingredients in a bowl.

3.   Make small meatballs from this mixture.

4.   Arrange the meatballs in a baking sheet and bake for 20 minutes.

5.   Cook all ingredients for the sauce for a few minutes.

6.   Serve the meatballs with sauce on top.

7.   Enjoy.

Preparation time: 10 minutes

Cooking time: 20 minutes

Total time: 30 minutes

Servings: 04

Nutritional Values:

- *Calories 334*
- *Total Fat 1.3 g*
- *Saturated Fat 5 g*
- *Cholesterol 31 mg*
- *Sodium 86 mg*
- *Total Carbs 8 g*
- *Fiber 2.3 g*
- *Sugar 2.2 g*
- *Protein 4.6 g*

Grilled Marinated Shrimp

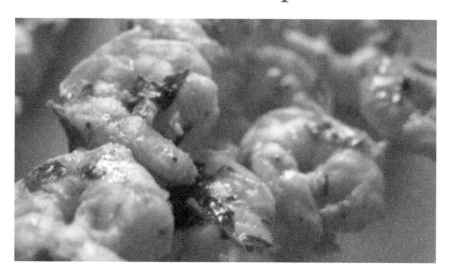

Ingredients:

- 1 cup vegetable oil
- 1/4 cup parsley chopped
- 3 cloves garlic, chopped
- 2 teaspoons dried oregano
- salt, to taste
- 1 teaspoon ground black pepper
- 2 pounds large shrimp, peeled and deveined with tails
- Attached skewers

How to prepare:

1. Combine parsley, with olive oil, lemon juice, garlic, oregano, salt, and black pepper.

2. Pour this marinade into a plastic bag while keeping some for basting.

3. Add shrimps to the plastic bag and marinate for 2 hours.
4. Meanwhile, preheat a grill and grease the grilling grates with olive oil.
5. Thread 2 to 3 shrimps on the skewers and grill them for 5 minutes per side while basting with the remaining marinade.
6. Serve.

Preparation time: 10 minutes

Cooking time: 15 minutes

Total time: 25 minutes

Servings: 04

Nutritional Values:

- *Calories 124*
- *Total Fat 3.5 g*
- *Saturated Fat 7 g*
- *Cholesterol 51 mg*
- *Sodium 86 mg*
- *Total Carbs 7.5 g*
- *Fiber 2.3 g*
- *Sugar 2.2 g*
- *Protein 14.5 g*

Japanese Chicken Wings

/

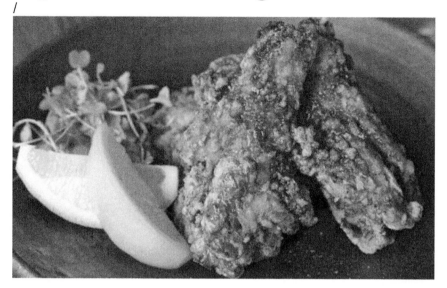

Ingredients:

- 3 pounds chicken wings
- 1 egg, lightly beaten
- 1 cup almond flour for coating
- 1 cup almond butter

Sauce

- 3 tablespoons coconut aminos
- 3 tablespoons water
- 1 cup coconut sugar
- 1/2 teaspoon garlic powder
- 1/2 cup apple cider vinegar
- 1 teaspoon salt

How to prepare:
1. Set the oven to 350 degrees F.
2. Slice the wings into half and dip them in the egg white whisk first.
3. Now coat the wings with almond flour.
4. Preheat the butter in a deep pan and stir fry the wings until golden brown.
5. Mix coconut aminos, garlic powder, salt, water, vinegar, and sweetener in a separate bowl.
6. Set the wings in a baking pan and pour the sauce over them.
7. Bake them for 20 minutes.
8. Serve.

Preparation time: 10 minutes

Cooking time: 20 minutes

Total time: 30 minutes

Servings: 06

Nutritional Values:
- *Calories 221*
- *Total Fat 12.4 g*
- *Saturated Fat 5 g*
- *Cholesterol 61 mg*
- *Sodium 216 mg*
- *Total Carbs 28 g*
- *Fiber 2.3 g*
- *Sugar 1.2 g*
- *Protein 7.6 g*

Baked Buffalo Wings

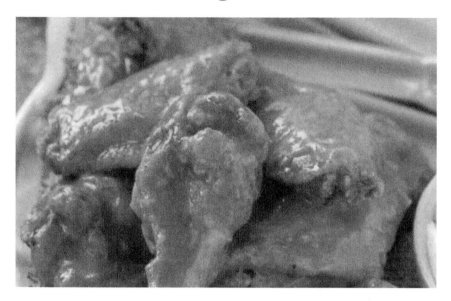

Ingredients:

- 3/4 cup almond flour
- ½ teaspoon onion powder
- 1/2 teaspoon garlic powder
- 1/2 teaspoon salt
- 20 chicken wings
- 1 cup melted almond butter

How to prepare:

1. Layer a baking sheet with tin foil and grease it with cooking spray.
2. Combine flour with garlic powder, onion powder, and salt in a plastic bag.
3. Shake this mixture then add the wings to the bag and seal.

4. Again, shake the wings to coat well then spread them onto a baking sheet.
5. Refrigerate them for 30 minutes.
6. Meanwhile, set the oven to 400 degrees F.
7. Dip the coated wings into the batter and then arrange them on a baking sheet.
8. Bake them for 45 minutes while flipping after 20 minutes.
9. Serve.

Preparation time: 10 minutes
Cooking time: 50 minutes
Total time: 60 minutes
Servings: 10

Nutritional Values:

- *Calories 153*
- *Total Fat 2.4 g*
- *Saturated Fat 3 g*
- *Cholesterol 21 mg*
- *Sodium 216 mg*
- *Total Carbs 8 g*
- *Fiber 2.3 g*
- *Sugar 1.2 g*
- *Protein 3.2 g*

Spinach Brownies

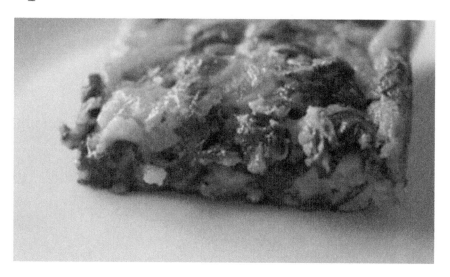

Ingredients:

- 1 (10 ounces) package spinach, rinsed and chopped
- 1 cup almond flour
- 1 teaspoon salt
- 1 teaspoon baking powder
- 2 egg whites
- 1 cup almond milk
- 1/2 cup almond butter, melted
- 1 onion, chopped
- 1 (8 ounces) package shredded mozzarella cheese

How to prepare:

1. Set the oven at 375 degrees F. Grease a 9x13 inch baking pan with cooking oil.

2. Spread the spinach in the saucepan and cover it with water.
3. Cook the spinach for 3 minutes and then immediately drain it.
4. Mix flour with salt and baking powder.
5. Add milk, butter, and egg. Whisk well and then add onion, spinach, and cheese.
6. Spread this mixture into the baking dish and bake for 30 minutes.
7. Slice and serve.

Preparation time: 10 minutes
Cooking time: 35 minutes
Total time: 45 minutes
Servings: 04

Nutritional Values:

- *Calories 454*
- *Total Fat 4 g*
- *Saturated Fat 5 g*
- *Cholesterol 0 mg*
- *Sodium 233 mg*
- *Total Carbs 30 g*
- *Fiber 6 g*
- *Sugar 2.2 g*
- *Protein 4 g*

VEGETARIAN AND VEGAN RECIPES

Pepper and Onion Tart

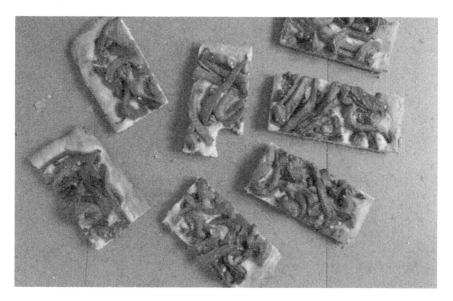

Ingredients:

- 2 tablespoon vegetable oil
- 2 onions, peeled and finely sliced
- 1 garlic clove, finely sliced
- 3 1/3 cup (1 sheet) ready-made puff pastry
- 2 cups red bell peppers, sliced
- 2 sprigs thyme
- 1-2 tablespoon apple cider vinegar
- salt
- pepper

How to prepare:

1. Set the oven to 400 degrees F.
2. Preheat a pan with oil and saute onions until golden and soft.
3. Stir in garlic and stir cook for 5 minutes.
4. Spread the puff pastry sheet on a lightly floured surface.
5. Place the sheet in a greased baking pan and score the edges around the rims.
6. Bake the crust for 5 minutes.
7. Add onions mixture over the pastry and top it with bell pepper.
8. Drizzle thyme leaves, apple cider vinegar, salt, and pepper.
9. Bake for 15 minutes at 400 degrees F.
10. Slice and serve.

Preparation time: 5 minutes

Cooking time: 20 minutes

Total time: 25 minutes

Servings: 04

Nutritional Values:

- *Calories 383*
- *Total Fat 5.3 g*
- *Saturated Fat 3.9 g*
- *Cholesterol 135 mg*
- *Sodium 487 mg*
- *Total Carbs 76.8 g*
- *Fibre 0.1g*
- *Sugar 0 g*
- *Protein 17.7 g*

Oat and Chickpea Dumplings

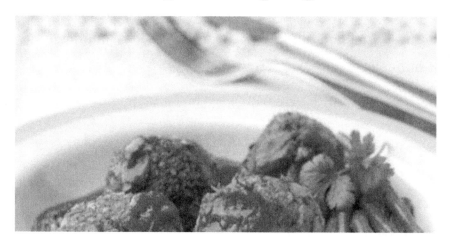

Ingredients:

- 6 tablespoon rapeseed oil
- 2 medium onions, finely chopped
- 2 teaspoon ground cumin
- 2 cans chickpeas, drained
- 1 pack coriander
- 1/2 cups oats
- 2 cups passata with onion and garlic

How to prepare:

1. Grease a frying pan with 2 tablespoon oil and sauté onions for 5 minutes until golden.
2. Stir in cumin and cook for 1 minute then keep the mixture in a food processor.
3. Add coriander, chickpeas, seasoning, and 2 tablespoons of oil. Blend until smooth.

4. Fold in oats and make 16 small balls from it.
5. Heat oil for frying and cook the dumpling for 3 minutes.
6. Stir in passata along with water and let it simmer for 2 minutes.
7. Serve warm.

Preparation time: 5 minutes

Cooking time: 15 minutes

Total time: 20 minutes

Servings: 4

Nutritional Values:

- *Calories 198*
- *Total Fat 3.8 g*
- *Saturated Fat 5.1 g*
- *Cholesterol 20 mg*
- *Sodium 272 mg*
- *Total Carbs 3.6 g*
- *Fiber 1 g*
- *Sugar 1.3 g*
- *Protein 1.8 g*

Mushroom risotto

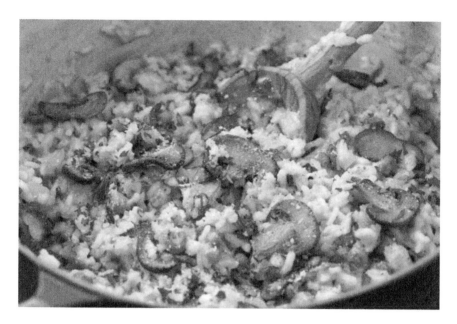

Ingredients:

- 2 tablespoons dried porcini mushrooms
- 1½ tablespoon olive oil
- 1 1/4 cup pack chestnut mushrooms, sliced
- 1 small onion, finely diced
- 1 garlic clove, crushed
- 1 1/6 cup Arborio rice
- 1/3 cup broth
- 1/2 cups baby spinach
- 1/4 cup feta, crumbled

How to prepare:

1. Add dried mushrooms to the boiled water and keep it aside.

2. Heat 1 tablespoon oil in a deep pan and sauté chestnut mushrooms for 5 minutes.

3. Keep the sautéed mushrooms aside.

4. Add ½ tablespoon oil more to the pan. Sauté garlic and onions for 6 minutes.

5. Strain dried mushrooms and chop them roughly.

6. Add mushrooms to the pan along with rice and broth.

7. Cook until the liquid is absorbed and then return the chestnut mushrooms to the mixture.

8. Add reserved mushroom liquid and continue cooking until all the liquid is absorbed.

9. Stir in spinach and cook for 2 minutes.

10. Serve.

Preparation time: 10 minutes

Cooking time: 20 minutes

Total time: 30 minutes

Servings: 2

Nutritional Values:

- *Calories 372*
- *Total Fat 11.8 g*
- *Saturated Fat 4.4 g*
- *Cholesterol 62 mg*
- *Sodium 871 mg*
- *Total Carbs 11.8 g*
- *Fiber 0.6 g*
- *Sugar 7.3 g*
- *Protein 4 g*

Spaghetti with watercress and pea pesto

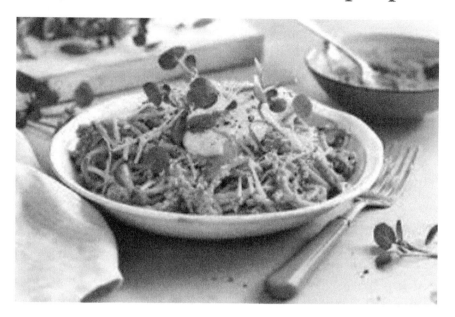

Ingredients:

- 2 cups frozen peas
- 2 garlic cloves
- 1/4 cup watercress
- 2 tablespoon hazelnuts, toasted
- 1/4 cup vegetarian hard cheese
- 2 tablespoons olive oil
- 3 1/4 cup whole meal spaghetti
- 4 egg whites

How to prepare:

1. Heat water to a simmer in a cooking pan and then add garlic and peas.
2. Cook for 3 minutes, drain, and then set it aside.

3. Blend peas with garlic, watercress, cheese, and hazelnuts until it forms into a thick paste.
4. Add olive oil and blend again until smooth.
5. Meanwhile, boil spaghetti as per the given instructions then drain and keep it aside.
6. Add water to a suitable cooking pot and bring it to simmer.
7. Create a whirlpool in the water and egg whites into it. Cook for 3 minutes.
8. Mix pesto with spaghetti and serve with poached egg whites, black pepper, and watercress on top.

Preparation time: 10 minutes
Cooking time: 30 minutes
Total time: 40 minutes
Servings: 4

Nutritional Values:

- *Calories 341*
- *Total Fat 4 g*
- *Saturated Fat 0.5 g*
- *Cholesterol 69 mg*
- *Sodium 547 mg*
- *Total Carbs 16.4 g*
- *Fiber 1.2 g*
- *Sugar 1 g*
- *Protein 0.3 g*

Vegetarian pasta bakes with halloumi

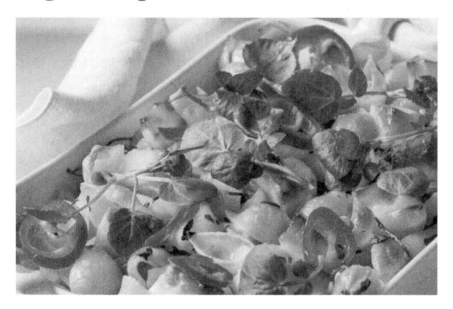

Ingredients:
- 2 cups conchiglie pasta
- 2 cups frozen broad beans
- 2/3 cup mascarpone
- 1/4 cup pack watercress
- 1 lemon, zested
- 2 x 1 1/6 cup packs chargrilled artichokes, thinly sliced
- 1 1/3 cup halloumi, cubed
- 1 large red chili, sliced (optional)

How to prepare:
1. Set the oven to 400 degrees F. Meanwhile boil salted water in a pan.
2. Add pasta to the water and cook for 10 minutes. Stir in broad beans.

3. Cook for 2 minutes then adds mascarpone.
4. Chop watercress and add it to the pasta, along with lemon zest and seasoning.
5. Spread half of the pasta mixture in a baking dish and top it with sliced artichokes.
6. Add the remaining half of the pasta. Top it with halloumi cubes.
7. Bake for 30 minutes.
8. Garnish as desired and serve.

Preparation time: 10 minutes
Cooking time: 40 minutes
Total time: 50 minutes
Servings: 04

Nutritional Values:
- *Calories 311*
- *Total Fat 0.5 g*
- *Saturated Fat 2.4 g*
- *Cholesterol 69 mg*
- *Sodium 58 mg*
- *Total Carbs 1.4 g*
- *Fiber 0.7 g*
- *Sugar 0.3 g*
- *Protein 1.4 g*

Broccoli pesto penne with chili and garlic

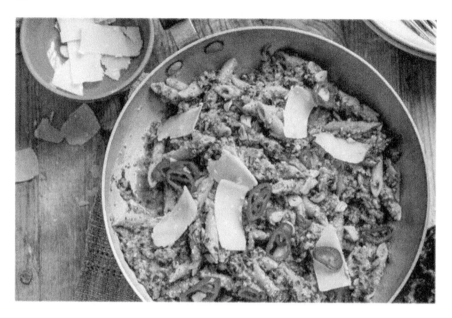

Ingredients:

- 1 1/4 cup whole wheat penne
- 2 cups broccoli florets
- 2 tablespoons basil
- 2 tablespoons flat-leaf parsley
- 2 teaspoons roasted chopped hazelnuts
- 3 teaspoon olive oil
- 2 tablespoons vegetarian hard cheese
- 2 garlic cloves, thinly sliced
- 1 large red chili, sliced into thin rounds

How to prepare:

1. Boil penne pasta as per the given instruction on the pack.
2. Blanch broccoli for 3 minutes in hot water and then drain.

3. Grind broccoli with parsley, basil, oil, and nuts in a processor.
4. Add cheese and 4 tablespoons of cooking water, along with seasoning, to the blender.
5. Drain the pasta and add it to a bowl while tossing with broccoli pesto.
6. Heat oil in a cooking pan and saute garlic with chilli for 1 minute.
7. Serve pasta with sauteed garlic mixture.
8. Garnish as desired.
9. Enjoy.

Preparation time: 10 minutes
Cooking time: 15 minutes
Total time: 25 minutes
Servings: 2

Nutritional Values:
- *Calories 304*
- *Total Fat 30.6 g*
- *Saturated Fat 13.1 g*
- *Cholesterol 131 mg*
- *Sodium 834 mg*
- *Total Carbs 21.4g*
- *Fiber 0.2 g*
- *Sugar 0.3 g*
- *Protein 4.6 g*

Veggie rice bowl

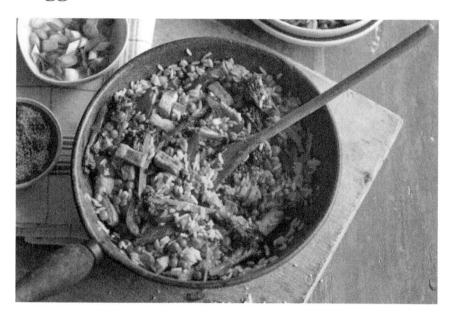

Ingredients:

- 1 tablespoon vegetable oil
- 1 ½ cup pack Tender stem broccoli tips, halved lengthways
- 1 red bell pepper, seeded and diced
- 1 1/4 cup pack marinated tofu pieces
- 2 x 2 1/4 cup pouches microwave rice
- 2 cups frozen peas
- 1 tablespoon sesame seeds
- 3 spring onions, chopped
- 1 garlic clove, crushed
- 2.5cm piece fresh ginger, grated
- 3 tablespoon coconut aminos
- 2 tablespoons sweet chili sauce
- 1 tablespoon apple cider vinegar

How to prepare:

1. Preheat oil in a cooking wok.

2. Sauté broccoli with pepper for 3 minutes.

3. Add diced tofu and cook for 2 minutes.

4. Stir in rice and stir cook for 4 minutes. Add peas to cook for another 3 minutes.

5. Make the sauce by mixing the sweet chili sauce with the garlic, coconut aminos, and vinegar.

6. Pour the sauce over the rice mixture and serve with spring onions and sesame seeds on top.

7. Enjoy.

Preparation time: 10 minutes

Cooking time: 20 minutes

Total time: 30 minutes

Servings: 04

Nutritional Values:

- *Calories 418*
- *Total Fat 3.8 g*
- *Saturated Fat 0.7 g*
- *Cholesterol 2 mg*
- *Sodium 620 mg*
- *Total Carbs 13.3 g*
- *Fiber 2.4 g*
- *Sugar 1.2 g*
- *Protein 5.4g*

Thai tofu and red cabbage bowl

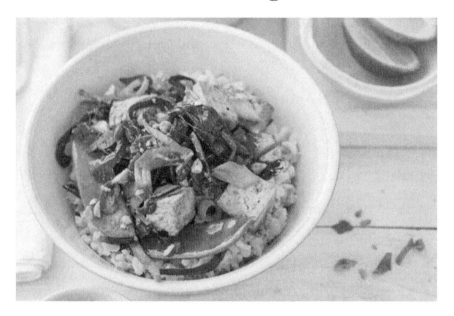

Ingredients:

- 2 cups (10oz) easy cook brown rice
- 1 stick lemongrass, halved lengthways
- For the tofu
- 2 tablespoon groundnut oil
- 3 ¼ cup tofu, cut into 2cm (1in) cubes
- 1 red bird's-eye chili, finely sliced
- 1/6 cup (1 1/2oz) pieces of ginger, sliced
- 2 cloves garlic, chopped
- 4 spring onions, sliced
- 1 lime, juiced
- 2 tablespoon coconut aminos
- 1/2 small red cabbage, sliced

- 1/2 cups (3 1/2oz) snap peas
- 2 tablespoons (1/2oz) basil leaves, sliced
- 4 tablespoon peanuts, toasted and roughly chopped, to serve
- 1 lime, quartered, to serve

How to prepare:
1. Add rice, lemon grass and 1 pt. water to a cooking pot.
2. Boil the rice then reduce the heat to cook for 25 minutes until al dente.
3. Meanwhile, heat oil in a wok and sauté tofu for 6 minutes.
4. Add garlic, spring onion, ginger, and chili. Stir cook for 1 minute.
5. Add coconut aminos and lime juice.
6. Stir in snap peas, and red cabbage. Cook for 3 minutes.
7. Add basil then put off the heat.
8. To serve, add rice to the serving bowl and then top them with the tofu mixture.
9. Garnish with peanuts.
10. Serve.

Preparation time: 10 minutes
Cooking time: 40 minutes
Total time: 50 minutes
Servings: 04

Nutritional Values:

- *Calories 438*
- *Total Fat 4.8 g*
- *Saturated Fat 1.7 g*
- *Cholesterol 12 mg*
- *Sodium 520 mg*
- *Total Carbs 58.3 g*
- *Fiber 2.3 g*
- *Sugar 1.2 g*
- *Protein 2.1 teaspoon*

Vegan shepherd's pie

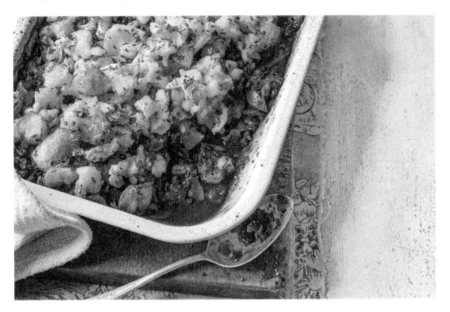

Ingredients:

- 3 2/3 cups miniature potatoes
- 2 tablespoons flat leaf parsley, finely chopped
- 3 tablespoon olive oil
- 1 onion, finely chopped
- 2 cups closed cup mushrooms, halved and thinly sliced
- 2 garlic cloves, finely chopped
- ¼ teaspoon crushed chilies
- 21/4 cup ready-to-eat puy lentils
- 2 cups chopped red bell pepper
- 2 tablespoon yogurt

How to prepare:

1. Boil potatoes for 15 minutes until al dente; then drain and return to the pot.

2. Crush the potatoes lightly while seasoning with spices and parsley.
3. Preheat 2 tablespoon oil in a deep pan. Saute onion for 3 minutes.
4. Increase the heat to saute mushrooms for 7 minutes.
5. Add chilies, garlic, puree, lentil, and water to the pot. Cook for 10 minutes.
6. Season the mixture and add parsley.
7. Preheat the grill on high heat.
8. Spread the mushroom mixture in a baking dish. Top it with crushed potatoes evenly.
9. Drizzle remaining oil and grill for 10 minutes.
10. Serve.

Preparation time: 10 minutes
Cooking time: 45 minutes
Total time: 55 minutes
Servings: 04

Nutritional Values:
- *Calories 246*
- *Total Fat 14.8 g*
- *Saturated Fat 0.7 g*
- *Cholesterol 22 mg*
- *Sodium 220 mg*
- *Total Carbs 40.3 g*
- *Fiber 2.4 g*
- *Sugar 1.2 g*
- *Protein 12.4g*

Vegan vegetable curry

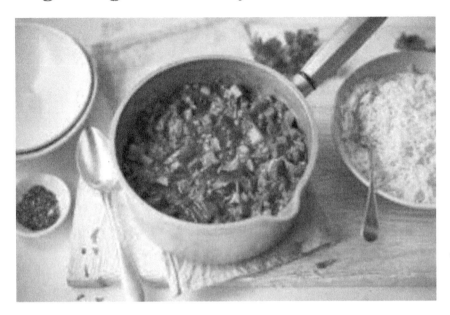

Ingredients:

- 1 tablespoon vegetable oil
- 1 large onion, finely chopped
- s5cm piece ginger, finely chopped
- 2 garlic cloves, finely chopped
- 1 teaspoon ground cumin
- 1 teaspoon ground coriander
- 1 teaspoon ground turmeric
- 1 aubergine, chopped into 1cm pieces
- 1 cup yogurt
- ½ cup vegetable stock
- 1 zucchini chopped into 1 cm pieces
- 1/2 cups spinach
- 1 1/4 cup peas (fresh or defrosted, if frozen)

How to prepare:

1. Preheat oil in a large cooking pan. Sauté onion for 7 minutes.
2. Add ginger and garlic to sauté for 3 minutes.
3. Stir in dried spices and chili. Cook for 1 minute.
4. Add aubergine, yogurt, and stock. Cook for 10 minutes.
5. Stir in zucchini and continue cooking with the closed lid for 25 minutes.
6. Uncover and cook for 10 minutes.
7. Add spinach and peas. Cook for 3 minutes.
8. Serve.

Preparation time: 10 minutes
Cooking time: 60 minutes
Total time: 1hr. 10 minutes
Servings: 04

Nutritional Values:

- *Calories 338*
- *Total Fat 3.8 g*
- *Saturated Fat 0.7 g*
- *Cholesterol 22 mg*
- *Sodium 620 mg*
- *Total Carbs 58.3 g*
- *Fiber 2.4 g*
- *Sugar 1.2 g*
- *Protein 5.4g*

SEAFOOD AND POULTRY RECIPES

Seafood paella recipe

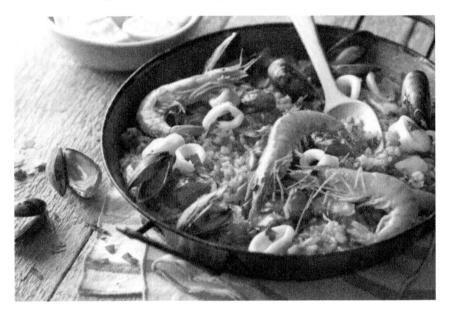

Ingredients:

- 1 1/2 pint fish stock
- pinch saffron
- 1 1/2 tablespoon extra-virgin olive oil
- 1 large onion, finely chopped
- 3 crushed garlic cloves
- 1 1/4oz pack, flatleaf parsley, leaves chopped
- 1 teaspoon black pepper
- 21/4 cup (8oz) Spanish paella rice
- 1 cup red bell pepper, chopped
- 1 x 21/4 cup jar roasted peppers, drain and rinse them

- 1 1/3 cup (6oz) raw black tiger prawns
- 1 1/4 cup (5oz) live mussels, cleaned and debearded
- 1 1/4 cup raw squid rings
- 1 lemon, cut into wedges

How to prepare:

1. Boil fish stock with saffron and keep it aside.
2. Preheat the oil to saute onion for 5 minutes.
3. Add garlic, bell pepper, parsley, and black pepper. Stir cook for 2 minutes.
4. Stir in rice, stock and cook for 10 minutes.
5. Add in roasted peppers and cook for 5 minutes.
6. Place prawns, mussels, and squid rings in the pan.
7. Cook for 5 mins then place off the heat.
8. Cover the pan with foil and let it sit for 5 minutes.
9. Garnish with parsley.
10. Serve.

Preparation time: 10 minutes

Cooking time: 40 minutes

Total time: 50 minutes

Servings: 4

Nutritional Values:

- *Calories 272*
- *Total Fat 11 g*
- *Saturated Fat 3 g*
- *Cholesterol 66 mg*
- *Sodium 288 mg*
- *Total Carbs 10 g*
- *Fibre 4g*
- *Sugar 0 g*
- *Protein 33 g*

Sicilian Seafood Stew

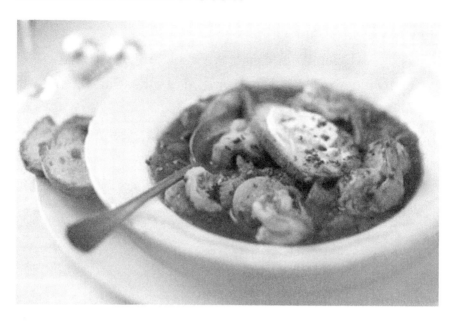

Ingredients:

- 2 tablespoon olive oil
- 1 onion, chopped
- 2 sticks celery, chopped
- 2 garlic cloves, chopped, plus an extra clove
- 1 anchovy, rinsed
- 1teaspoon dried chili flakes
- 1 cup red bell pepper
- ½ cup nonfat yogurt
- 2 cups vegetable stock
- 3 cups raw peeled prawns
- 2 cups new potatoes
- zest and juice of 1 lemon
- 1 teaspoon baby capers
- 1 teaspoon flat leaf parsley, chopped

How to prepare:

1. Preheat olive oil in a suitable pot and sauté celery, onion, anchovy, garlic, and chili.

2. Season with pepper and salt. Stir cook for 5 mins.

3. Meanwhile, boil potatoes until al dente. Cut them into thick slices.

4. Add stock, yogurt and bell pepper to the pan and cook for 15 minutes.

5. Place prawns in the pan along with potatoes, capers, lemon zest, and juice.

6. Cook for 5 mins then serve.

Preparation time: 10 minutes
Cooking time: 25 minutes
Total time: 35 minutes
Servings: 4

Nutritional Values:

- *Calories 557*
- *Total Fat 29 g*
- *Saturated Fat 22 g*
- *Cholesterol 550 mg*
- *Sodium 1800 mg*
- *Total Carbs 25 g*
- *Fiber 3 g*
- *Sugar 0.3 g*
- *Protein 47 g*

Seafood stew

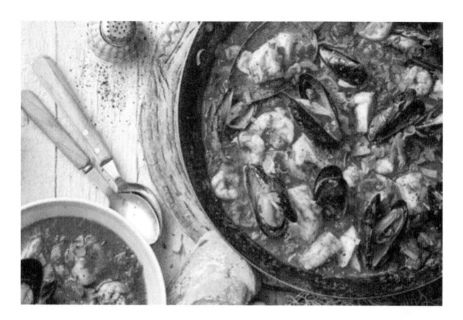

Ingredients:

- 1 large onion, finely sliced
- 1 garlic clove, finely chopped
- Black pepper, to taste
- 1 cup nonfat yogurt
- 2 cups chicken stock
- 41/4 cup skinless white fish fillets, chopped into large chunks
- 11/3 cup raw peeled king prawns
- 2 cups mussels, cleaned and debearded
- small bunch flat-leaf parsley leaves roughly chopped
- crusty bread and almond butter, to serve (optional)

How to prepare:

1. Preheat oil in a pan and saute for onions for 5 minutes.
2. Add pepper and garlic, stir cook for 2 minutes.
3. Pour in stock and yogurt. Cook for 10 minutes.
4. Place fish chunks in the pan and cook for 2 minutes.
5. Stir in mussels and prawns. Cover the pan and cook for 3 minutes.
6. Garnish with parsley.
7. Serve.

Preparation time: 05 minutes

Cooking time: 20 minutes

Total time: 25 minutes

Servings: 4

Nutritional Values:

- *Calories 301*
- *Total Fat 12.2 g*
- *Saturated Fat 2.4 g*
- *Cholesterol 110 mg*
- *Sodium 276 mg*
- *Total Carbs 5 g*
- *Fiber 0.9 g*
- *Sugar 1.4 g*
- *Protein 28.8 g*

Fritto Misto with gremolata

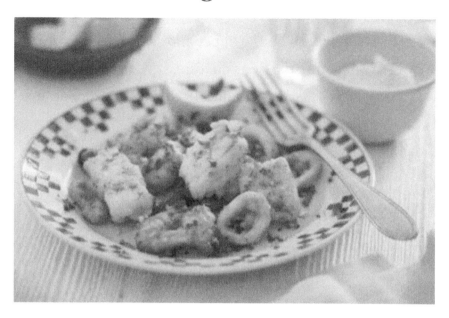

Ingredients:

- small bunch flat leaf parsley, finely chopped
- zest 1 lemon
- ½teaspoon garlic , finely chopped
- For the fritto Misto
- 1/3 cup (3oz) almond flour
- ¼teaspoon black pepper
- 21/4 cup cod fillet, bones removed and cut into bite-sized pieces
- 1 1/3 cup mixed seafood
- 6 tablespoon olive oil
- good quality mayo to serve

How to prepare:

1. Mix all the ingredients for gremolata.
2. Combine flour with black pepper and seasoning in a bowl.
3. Dip the seafood in the flour mixture.
4. Preheat oil in a frying pan and fry the coated seafood until golden brown.
5. Serve.

Preparation time: 5 minutes

Cooking time: 15 minutes

Total time: 20 minutes

Servings: 4

Nutritional Values:

- *Calories 310*
- *Total Fat 2.4 g*
- *Saturated Fat 0.1 g*
- *Cholesterol 320 mg*
- *Sodium 350 mg*
- *Total Carbs 12.2 g*
- *Fiber 0.7 g*
- *Sugar 0.7 g*
- *Protein 44.3 g*

Fritto Misto

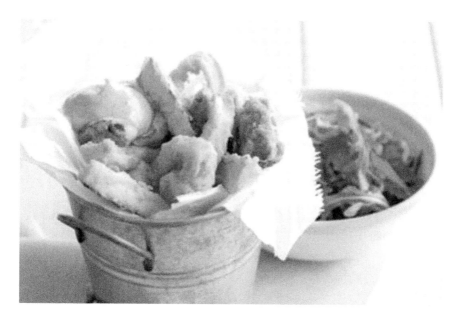

Ingredients:

- vegetable oil for deep frying
- 1 egg
- 1/2 pint whole milk
- 1lb mixed raw seafood, cut into pieces
- 1 zucchini, cut into batons
- 2/3 cup (4oz) almond flour
- 6 tablespoon cornflour
- 2/3 cup (4oz) semolina

How to prepare:

1. Preheat the oil to 320 degrees F in a deep pan.
2. Beat milk with egg white and seasonings.

3. Add seafood and zucchini to the milk.
4. Combine cornflour, semolina, and flour in a bowl.
5. Dip the seafood and zuchini in the flour mixture and shake off the excess.
6. Add oil to a deep and heat to fry until golden.
7. Serve.

Preparation time: 5 minutes

Cooking time: 10 minutes

Total time: 15 minutes

Servings: 2

Nutritional Values:

- *Calories 372*
- *Total Fat 1.1 g*
- *Saturated Fat 3.8 g*
- *Cholesterol 10 mg*
- *Sodium 749 mg*
- *Total Carbs 4.9 g*
- *Fiber 0.2 g*
- *Sugar 0.2 g*
- *Protein 33.5 g*

Fish soup

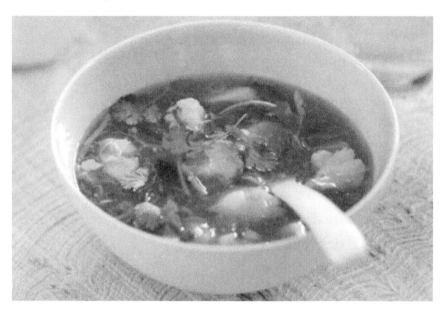

Ingredients:

- olive oil
- 2 small onions, finely chopped
- 2 carrots, finely chopped
- 2 celery stalks, finely chopped
- 4 garlic cloves, finely chopped
- 1-2 sweet peppers, deseeded and finely chopped
- 2½pt vegetable stock
- 4 cups fish stock
- 2 anchovy fillets in oil, drained
- salt
- pepper
- 21/4 cup (8oz) monkfish tail, all bones removed and flesh cut into cubes
- 21/4 cup (8oz) frozen seafood, defrosted and rinsed

- 2 handfuls small soup pasta
- handful olives (black or green), de-pitted and finely chopped
- fresh crusty bread, to serve

How to prepare:
1. Preheat olive oil in the pan and sauté onions, celery, peppers, and garlic until golden.
2. Stir in stock, anchovy, and pepper.
3. Cover the lid and cook for 40 minutes.
4. Stir in monkfish tail, pasta, and seafood.
5. Cover and cook for 20 minutes.
6. Serve with olives on top.
7. Enjoy.

Preparation time: 5 minutes
Cooking time: 15 minutes
Total time: 20 minutes
Servings: 2

Nutritional Values:
- *Calories 581*
- *Total Fat 23 g*
- *Saturated Fat 4 g*
- *Cholesterol 49 mg*
- *Sodium 257 mg*
- *Total Carbs 3.6g*
- *Fiber 10 g*
- *Sugar 0.5 g*
- *Protein 58 g*

Chicken Chasseur

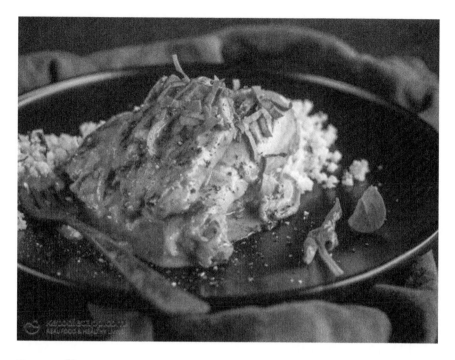

Ingredients:

- 4 chicken legs
- 1 tablespoon olive oil
- 1 onion, finely sliced
- 2 garlic cloves, finely sliced
- 2 1/4 cup (8oz) chestnut mushrooms, cut into 4 if small and 6 if large
- 3 1/2 cup chicken stock
- 1 bay leaf
- 1 thyme sprig
- 1 cup nonfat yogurt
- 1 red bell pepper, chopped
- small handful of tarragon, chopped

- mashed potatoes, to serve

How to prepare:
1. Sear chicken legs in some oil until golden brown.
2. Remove the chicken and saute onion until soft.
3. Add mushrooms and garlic until golden.
4. Stir in nonfatt yogurt, bay leaf, thyme, red bell pepper and chicken stock.
5. Boil the mixture and then reduce it to a simmer. Add chicken legs.
6. Cook for 30 minutes and add tarragon.
7. Serve.

Preparation time: 5 minutes
Cooking time: 30 minutes
Total time: 35 minutes
Servings: 04

Nutritional Values:
- *Calories 529*
- *Total Fat 17 g*
- *Saturated Fat 3 g*
- *Cholesterol 65 mg*
- *Sodium 391 mg*
- *Total Carbs 55 g*
- *Fiber 6 g*
- *Sugar 8 g*
- *Protein 41g*

Smoky chicken traybake

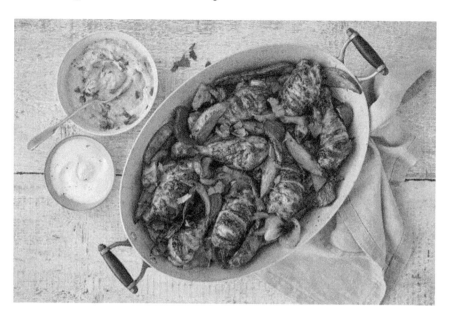

Ingredients:

- 2 lbs. pack chicken thighs and drumsticks
- olive oil, for greasing
- 1 red bell pepper, deseeded and roughly chopped
- 2 yellow bell peppers, deseeded and roughly chopped
- 2 red onions, peeled and sliced intoo wedges
- 1/2 cups barbecue sauce
- 7 1/4 cup sweet potatoes, scrubbed and cut into wedges
- 2/3 cup sour cream
- coriander leaves, to garnish
- guacamole, to serve

How to prepare:

1. Set the oven to 400degreese F. Score the skin of thethighss.

2. Place them with peppers and red onion in the roasting pan.

3. Mix all the remaining ingredients.

4. Top the chicken and vegetables with this paste.

5. Roast the chicken for 15 minutes then add sweet potato.

6. Turn all the drumsticks and bake for 30 minutes.

7. Serve.

Preparation time: 10 minutes

Cooking time: 45 minutes

Total time: 55 minutes

Servings: 4

Nutritional Values:

-   *Calories 284*
-   *Total Fat 25 g*
-   *Saturated Fat 1 g*
-   *Cholesterol 49 mg*
-   *Sodium 460 mg*
-   *Total Carbs 35 g*
-   *Fiber 2 g*
-   *Sugar 6 g*
-   *Protein 26g*

Chicken and Orzo Bake

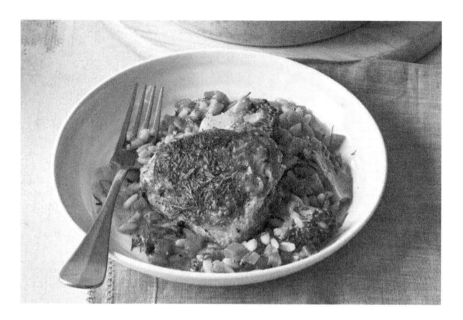

Ingredients:

- ½ tablespoon olive oil
- 4 bone-in chicken thighs, from a 1kg pack
- 2 onions, finely chopped
- 2 celery sticks, finely chopped
- 1 carrot, peeled and finely chopped
- 1 garlic clove, finely chopped
- 1 teaspoon fennel seeds
- 2 cups orzo
- 1 chicken stock cube, made up with 2 cups hot water
- 2 cups frozen broccoli florets
- handful of fresh dill, chopped
- 1 lemon, cut into wedges to serve

How to prepare:

1. Preheat the oil in a deep cooking pan.
2. Season the chicken and stir cook for 5 minutes per side.
3. Remove the chicken from the cooking pan and keep it aside.
4. Drain the excess fat and keep it aside.
5. Add onion, carrot, celery, garlic, and fennel seeds to the pan.
6. Stir cook for 10 minutes then add stock and orzo.
7. Return the chicken to the pan.
8. Boil the mixture and cook for 5 minutes on simmer.
9. Add broccoli and cook for 20 minutes.
10. Garnish with dill, and pepper.
11. Serve.

Preparation time: 5 minutes
Cooking time: 35 minutes
Total time: 40 minutes
Servings: 4

Nutritional Values:
- *Calories 152*
- *Total Fat 4 g*
- *Saturated Fat 2 g*
- *Cholesterol 65 mg*
- *Sodium 220 mg*
- *Total Carbs 1 teaspoon*
- *Fiber 0 g*
- *Sugar 1 g*
- *Protein 26g*

One-Pot Roast

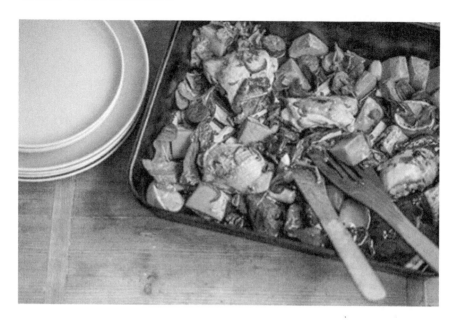

Ingredients:

- 8 Chicken thighs
- 1½lbs. sweet potato, cut into chunks
- 2 cups (7oz) chorizo sausage, sliced
- 1 bulb garlic, broken into cloves
- 2 tablespoon Grapeseed oil
- 1/3 cup chicken stock
- 1 lemon, halved
- 2 zucchinis, cut into thick batons
- 1 red chili, deseeded and sliced
- 2 1/6 cup (8oz) baby spinach
- 2 tablespoon parsley, chopped
- 1 pinch salt
- 1 pinch black pepper

How to prepare:

1. Set the oven to 400 degrees F.
2. Place chicken with sweet potato in a roasting pan.
3. Top the chicken with garlic, grapeseed oil, stock and lemon juice.
4. Bake for 50 minutes. Add zucchini, chili, and chorizo after 30 mins of baking.
5. Garnish with parsley and spinach.
6. Serve.

Preparation time: 10 minutes

Cooking time: 50 minutes

Total time: 60 minutes

Servings: 8

Nutritional Values:

- *Calories 188*
- *Total Fat 8 g*
- *Saturated Fat 1 g*
- *Cholesterol 0 mg*
- *Sodium 339 mg*
- *Total Carbs 8 g*
- *Fiber 1 g*
- *Sugar 2 g*
- *Protein 13g*

BEEF AND LAMB RECIPES

Beef curry

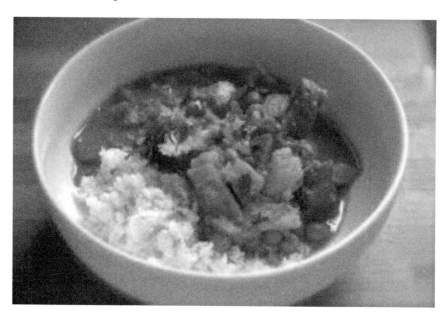

Ingredients:

- 14oz. beef rump, sliced thinly
- 1/4 cup sunflower oil
- 1 cup brown rice
- 41/4 cup boiling water
- 1 tablespoon fresh ginger, minced
- a few slices of fresh ginger
- 2 cloves garlic, minced
- 1 teaspoon ground cumin
- 1 teaspoon ground coriander
- 1 teaspoon turmeric

- 1 teaspoon ground black pepper
- ½ teaspoon chilli powder
- ½ teaspoon ground ginger
- 1/2 cups frozen peas
- sprigs of coriander, to garnish
- salt

How to prepare:

1. Boill rice in salted water and cook for 12 minutes. Drain and keep aside.
2. Preheat sunflower oil inthe pan and sear the beef until brown.
3. Remove the beef to the plate lined with a paper towel.
4. Add ginger and garlic, saute for few minutes.
5. Stir in spices and water.
6. Cook for 10 minutes then add peas.
7. Adjust seasoning and garnish with coriander.
8. Serve.

Preparation time: 10 minutes

Cooking time: 25 minutes

Total time: 35 minutes

Servings: 4

Nutritional Values:

- Calories 301
- Total Fat 15.8 g
- Saturated Fat 2.7 g
- Cholesterol 75 mg
- Sodium 1189 mg
- Total Carbs 11.7 g
- Fibre 0.3g
- Sugar 0.1 g
- Protein 28.2 g

Beef schnitzel

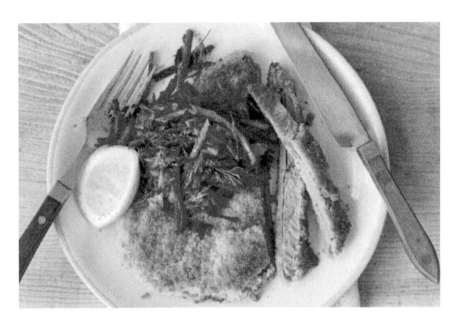

Ingredients:

- 4 tablespoon almond flour
- 1 large egg, beaten
- 1 1/4 cup (5oz) breadcrumbs
- 2 x 3 1/6 cup beef medallion steaks
- 2 tablespoon olive oil
- 1 lemon, cut into wedges to serve

For the slaw

- 2 raw beetroot, peeled and grated
- 1 large carrot, peeled and grated
- 1/2 red onion, peeled and finely sliced

- 2 stalks celery, finely sliced
- 1/2 pack dill, leaves chopped
- 1 lemon, juiced and zested
- 1 tablespoon extra-virgin olive oil

How to prepare:

1. Combine everything for the slaw in a bowl. Adjust seasoning with salt.
2. Mix flour with lemon zest and salt.
3. Beat egg white in a bowl and spread breadcrumbs in a shallow bowl.
4. Place each beef medallion in between 2 sheets of parchment paper.
5. Pound the meat using a rolling pin to reduce the thickness.
6. First dip the meat into the flour mixture; then add the egg and then breadcrumbs.
7. Preheat oil in a frying pan and cook the coated meat for 2 minutes per side.
8. Serve with slaw.

Preparation time: 10 minutes

Cooking time: 30 minutes

Total time: 40 minutes

Servings: 6

Nutritional Values:

- *Calories 308*
- *Total Fat 20.5 g*
- *Saturated Fat 3 g*
- *Cholesterol 0 mg*
- *Sodium 688 mg*
- *Total Carbs 10.3 g*
- *Sugar 1.4g*
- *Fiber 4.3 g*
- *Protein 49 g*

Beef Massaman Curry

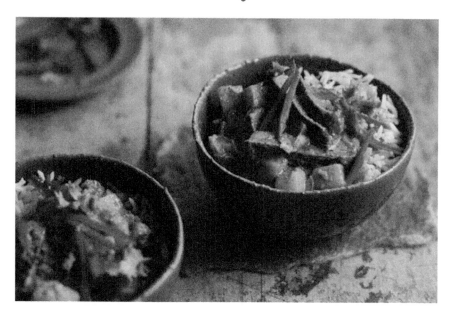

Ingredients:

- 1½ tablespoon vegetable oil
- 2 onions, chopped
- 21/4 cup Thai jasmine rice
- 2 cup Thai Massaman paste
- 3 cups potatoes, cut into 2cm-thick slices
- 51/4 cup cooked roast beef, cut into chunks
- 11/3 cup pack baby corn and snap peas,

How to prepare:

1. Preheat oil in a deep-frying pan and sauté onions for 10 minutes on low heat.

2. Boil rice in salted water for 10 minutes then drain and keep them aside.

3. Add Massaman paste and cook for 1 minute.

4. Put in sliced potato, coconut milk and star anise.

5. Cook this mixture for 15 minutes.

6. Add snap peas, a splash of water, corn, and beef.

7. Cook for 5 mins then serve.

Preparation time: 10 minutes

Cooking time: 30 minutes

Total time: 40 minutes

Servings: 6

Nutritional Values:

- *Calories 231*
- *Total Fat 20.1 g*
- *Saturated Fat 2.4 g*
- *Cholesterol 110 mg*
- *Sodium 941 mg*
- *Total Carbs 20.1 g*
- *Fiber 0.9 g*
- *Sugar 1.4 g*
- *Protein 14.6 g*

Barbecued rump of beef in Dijon

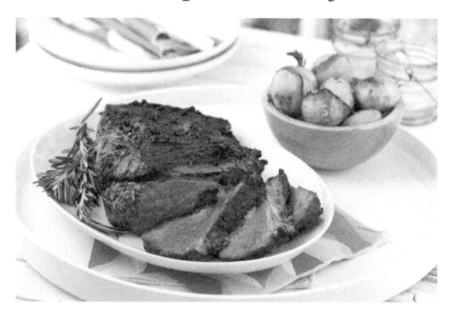

Ingredients:

- 2lbs. beef top rump joint
- 2 tablespoon fresh tarragon, roughly chopped
- 2 teaspoon black pepper
- 1 tablespoon Dijon mustard
- 2 tablespoons olive oil

How to prepare:

1. Keep the meat in a shallow dish and toss with tarragon, mustard, oil, and pepper to season.
2. Marinate the meat for 1.5 hours in the refrigerator.
3. Preheat the grill and grill for 15 minutes.
4. Carve and serve.

Preparation time: 10 minutes

Cooking time: 15 minutes

Total time: 25 minutes

Servings: 4

Nutritional Values:

- *Calories 280*
- *Total Fat 3.5 g*
- *Saturated Fat 0.1 g*
- *Cholesterol 320 mg*
- *Sodium 350 mg*
- *Total Carbs 7.6 g*
- *Fiber 0.7 g*
- *Sugar 0.7 g*
- *Protein 11.2 g*

Roast rib of beef

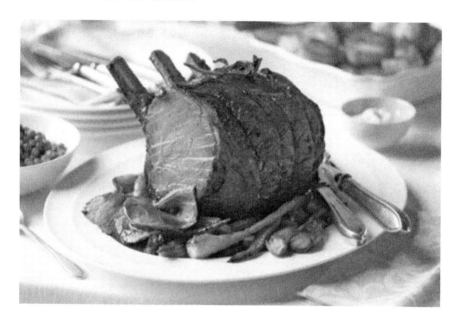

Ingredients:

- 2 Knorr Beef Stock Cubes
- 1 tablespoon olive oil
- 3lbs. rib of beef
- 5 small leeks
- 6 parsnips, peeled and halved
- 6 carrots, peeled and halved
- 4 shallots, peeled and halved
- celery sticks cut into large chunks
- fresh sage leaves

How to prepare:

1. Set the oven to 400 degrees F.
2. Mix 1 Knorr beef cube with 1 tablespoon oil and rub this paste onto the beef.
3. Sear the beef in a greased pan until brown then transfer them to a roasting pan.
4. Sauté leeks in the same pan until golden and place them around the beef.
5. Now sauté carrots and parsnips in the pan and also transfer them to the roasting pan.
6. Top the beef with sage, celery, and shallots.
7. Bake for 45 minutes.
8. Serve.

Preparation time: 10 minutes

Cooking time: 45 minutes

Total time: 55 minutes

Servings: 6

Nutritional Values:

- *Calories 472*
- *Total Fat 11.1 g*
- *Saturated Fat 5.8 g*
- *Cholesterol 610 mg*
- *Sodium 749 mg*
- *Total Carbs 19.9 g*
- *Fiber 0.2 g*
- *Sugar 0.2 g*
- *Protein 13.5 g*

Beef Wellington with Stilton

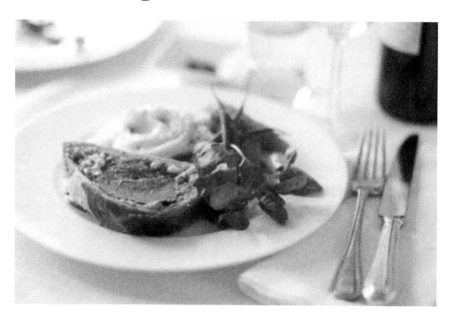

Ingredients:

- 2 tablespoon olive oil
- 2 tablespoons pine nuts
- 1 clove garlic, crushed
- 4 tablespoon horseradish sauce
- 1/4 cup (2oz) mature stilton, crumbled
- 1oz. fresh white breadcrumbs
- 1.5 lbs. piece of beef fillet
- 31/3 cup (13oz) ready rolled puff pastry
- beaten egg to glaze

How to prepare:

1. Preheat 1 tablespoon of oil in a frying pan and sauté pine nuts for 1 minute.

2. Toss in garlic and set the mixture aside to cool.
3. Combine stilton, horseradish, breadcrumbs, black pepper, and pine nuts mixture.
4. Heat more oil in a pan and sear beef fillet for 3 minutes per side until brown.
5. Adjust the oven to 400 degrees F.
6. Top the beef with horseradish mixture.
7. Spread the pastry sheet and top the beef pan with it.
8. Brush the pastry with beaten egg white.
9. Seal the edges and bake for 40 minutes.
10. Serve.

Preparation time: 5 minutes

Cooking time: 55 minutes

Total time: 60 minutes

Servings: 4

Nutritional Values:

- *Calories 327*
- *Total Fat 3.5 g*
- *Saturated Fat 0.5 g*
- *Cholesterol 162 mg*
- *Sodium 142 mg*
- *Total Carbs 33.6g*
- *Fiber 0.4 g*
- *Sugar 0.5 g*
- *Protein 24.5 g*

Marinated lamb steaks

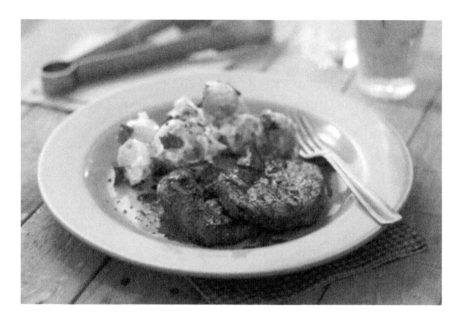

Ingredients:

- 6 lamb leg steaks
- 1/2 cup dark coconut aminos
- 1 tablespoon curry powder
- 1 teaspoon ground ginger
- 1tablespoon nonfat yogurt
- 1tablespoon olive oil
- salt
- pepper
- 2 cups new potatoes
- 2/3 cup pot natural yogurt
- 1 bunch mint
- 1 bunch spring onions

How to prepare:

1. Combine everything for the marinade and rub it over the lamb steaks.
2. Let it marinate for 1hour at room temperature.
3. Meanwhile, boil the potatoes in the salted water, drain them, and let them cool down.
4. Mix yogurt with spring onion and mint.
5. Toss in potatoes and seasonings.
6. Preheat grill and grill the lamb steaks for 3 minutes per side.
7. Serve with potatoes mixture.

Preparation time: 10 minutes
Cooking time: 30 minutes
Total time: 40 minutes
Servings: 6

Nutritional Values:

- *Calories 413*
- *Total Fat 7.5 g*
- *Saturated Fat 1.1 g*
- *Cholesterol 20 mg*
- *Sodium 97 mg*
- *Total Carbs 41.4 g*
- *Fiber 0 g*
- *Sugar 0 g*
- *Protein 21.1g*

Lamb kofta curry

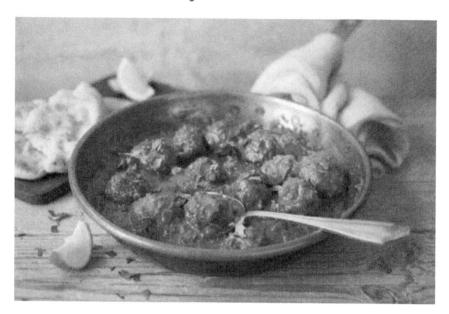

Ingredients:

- 2 tablespoon olive oil
- 2 red onions, finely chopped
- 3-4 long green chili peppers, deseeded, finely chopped
- 4 garlic cloves, chopped
- 5cm piece root ginger, grated
- 2 teaspoon ground cumin
- 1 teaspoon turmeric
- 1 teaspoon ground coriander
- 2 cups minced lamb
- ½ cup fine fresh white breadcrumbs
- 2 tablespoon chopped coriander
- 1 egg, beaten

- 2 teaspoon Panch Phoron seasoning
- 2 cups non-fat yogurt
- 1 cup hot vegetable stock
- 2 bay leaves
- 4 tablespoon coconut cream

How to prepare:

1. Preheat the grill on the medium heat.
2. Heat oil in suitable frying pan and sauté ginger, garlic, onions and chili for 5 minutes.
3. Reserve half of this mixture and add turmeric, coriander ground, and cumin.
4. Cook for 1 minute then remove it from the heat.
5. Mix minced meat with coriander, egg, and breadcrumbs.
6. Toss in onion mix and make small balls from this mixture.
7. Arrange the lamb meatballs in the baking dish and grill for 15 minutes.
8. Make the sauce by mixing onion mixture and Panch phiran. Cook for 2 minutes.
9. Add yogurt, stock, seasoning, and bay leaves. Cook for 15 minutes.
10. Discard the bay leaves and stir in coconut cream.

11. Blend the mixture then add meatballs. Cook for 10 minutes.
12. Serve.

Preparation time: 10 minutes

Cooking time: 50 minutes

Total time: 60 minutes

Servings: 4

Nutritional Values:

- *Calories 253*
- *Total Fat 7.5 g*
- *Saturated Fat 1.1 g*
- *Cholesterol 20 mg*
- *Sodium 297 mg*
- *Total Carbs 10.4 g*
- *Fiber 0 g*
- *Sugar 0 g*
- *Protein 13.1g*

Mediterranean Lamb Stew with Olives

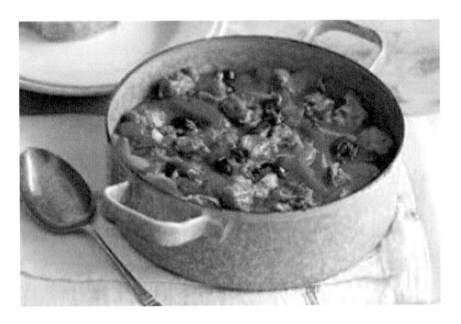

Ingredients:

- ½ lb. lamb leg steaks, cut into 2½ cm/ 1in chunks
- 1 cup yogurt, plus 4 tablespoons to serve
- 1 tablespoon medium curry powder
- 2 teaspoon cold-pressed rapeseed oil
- 2 medium onions, 1 thinly sliced, 1 cut into 5 wedges
- 2 garlic cloves, peeled and finely sliced
- 1 tablespoon ginger, peeled and finely chopped
- ¼ cup dried split red lentils, rinsed
- ½ small pack of coriander, roughly chopped, plus extra to garnish
- 1 cup pack baby leaf spinach

How to prepare:

1. Add oil to a suitable pan and heat.
2. Sear lamb for 10 minutes until brown. Transfer it to a plate lined with pepper.
3. Heat more oil and sauté onion for 5 minutes.
4. Stir in garlic and cook for 30 secs.
5. Return the lamb to the pan.
6. Add thyme, ¾ cup water, and orange peel.
7. Let it cook for 1 hour on a low simmer.
8. Stir in olives. Cook for 20 minutes then serve.

Preparation time: 15 minutes

Cooking time: 1 hr. 30 minutes

Total time: 1 hr. 35 minutes

Servings: 4

Nutritional Values:

- *Calories 201*
- *Total Fat 5.5 g*
- *Saturated Fat 2.1 g*
- *Cholesterol 10 mg*
- *Sodium 597 mg*
- *Total Carbs 2.4 g*
- *Fiber 0 g*
- *Sugar 0 g*
- *Protein 3.1g*

Herb and spiced lamb

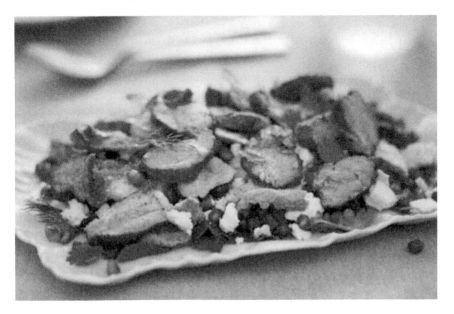

Ingredients:

- 14oz. lamb neck fillet, trimmed of sinew and excess fat
- ½ tablespoon cumin
- ½ tablespoon ground coriander
- 1 tablespoon toasted coriander seed, bashed
- 2 tablespoon olive oil, plus a drizzle
- 1 bunch mint, leaves picked
- 1 bunch dill, chopped
- 1 bunch coriander, leaves picked
- 2 cups feta
- 1 pomegranate, seeds only
- juice 1 lemon

How to prepare:

1. Set the oven to 400 degrees F.
2. Season, the lamb with the spices.
3. Heat oil in a suitable frying pan and sear the lamb for 3 minutes per side.
4. Place it in a baking sheet and roast for 10 minutes in the oven.
5. Top the lamb with remaining ingredients and serve.

Preparation time: 10 minutes

Cooking time: 20 minutes

Total time: 30 minutes

Servings: 4

Nutritional Values:

- *Calories 413*
- *Total Fat 8.5 g*
- *Saturated Fat 3.1 g*
- *Cholesterol 120 mg*
- *Sodium 497 mg*
- *Total Carbs 21.4 g*
- *Fiber 0.6 g*
- *Sugar 0.1 g*
- *Protein 14.1g*

SNACK AND SWEETS RECIPES

Mini pea pancakes

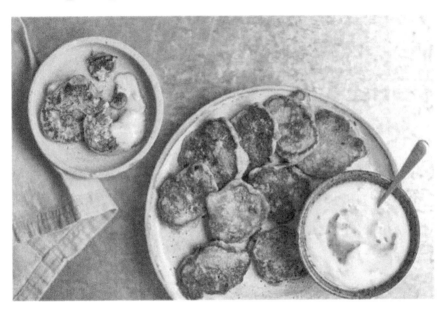

Ingredients:

- ¼ cup wholewheat flour
- ¼ cup almond flour
- 1½ teaspoon baking powder
- 3 egg whites
- 2 cups butter milk
- 1 1/4 cup frozen peas, defrosted
- sunflower oil spray, for frying

How to prepare:

1. Combine flour and baking powder in a bowl.
2. Whisk egg whites with buttermilk and 1/3 cup water.
3. Stir in flour mixture and mix well.
4. Fold in peas and keep the mixture aside.
5. Preheat a greased frying pan and add flour batter spoon by spoon.
6. Cook them for 2 minutes per side.
7. Serve.

Preparation time: 5 minutes
Cooking time: 15 minutes
Total time: 20 minutes
Servings: 4

Nutritional Values:

- *Calories 252*
- *Total Fat 16 g*
- *Saturated Fat 7 g*
- *Cholesterol 11 mg*
- *Sodium 8 mg*
- *Total Carbs 29 g*
- *Sugar 1.8 g*
- *Fiber 5 g*
- *Protein 4 g*

Halloumi Fries

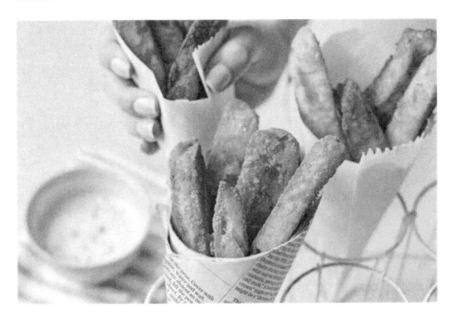

Ingredients:

- 1/3 cup (2 1/2oz) almond flour
- Salt to taste
- Black pepper to taste
- 2 x 9oz. packs halloumi, cut into chips
- sunflower oil, for frying
- 2 tablespoon chopped coriander

How to prepare:

1. Combine flour with seasonings and dip halloumi to coat.
2. Heat cooking oil in a deep pan until it sizzles.
3. Fry the coated halloumi for 2 minutes until golden brown.

4. Place the fries in a plate lined with paper towels.

5. Serve with coriander on top.

Preparation time: 10 minutes

Cooking time: 15 minutes

Total time: 25 minutes

Servings: 4

Nutritional Values:

- *Calories 386*
- *Total Fat 24 g*
- *Saturated Fat 3 g*
- *Cholesterol 0 mg*
- *Sodium 19 mg*
- *Total Carbs 41 g*
- *Sugar 1.9 g*
- *Fiber 7 g*
- *Protein 8 g*

Carrot Cupcakes

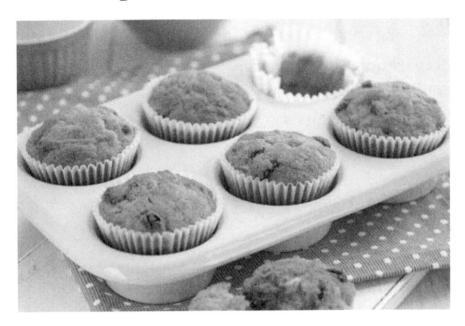

Ingredients:

- For the cupcakes
- 3 medium carrots, peeled and grated
- 1/2 cup coconut sugar
- ¼ cup almond butter, softened
- ¼ cup Golden syrup
- 2 medium egg whites
- 1 1/4 cup almond flour
- ½ teaspoon bicarbonate of soda
- 1 teaspoon ground cinnamon
- pinch of salt

How to prepare:

1. Adjust the oven to 375 degrees F. Layer a muffin tray with muffin cups.
2. Combine butter with golden syrup and sweetener in a suitable saucepan.
3. Cook for 2-3 minutes and then turn off the heat.
4. Stir in flour, soda, cinnamon, carrot, egg, and salt. Mix well until smooth.
5. Divide the batter into the muffin cups. Bake for 25 minutes.
6. Serve.

Preparation time: 15 minutes

Cooking time: 30 minutes

Total time: 45 minutes

Servings: 4

Nutritional Values:

- *Calories 190*
- *Total Fat 6 g*
- *Saturated Fat 2 g*
- *Cholesterol 2 mg*
- *Sodium 244 mg*
- *Total Carbs 31 g*
- *Sugar 3.6 g*
- *Fiber 0.8 g*
- *Protein 3 g*

Giant Chocolate Chip Cookie

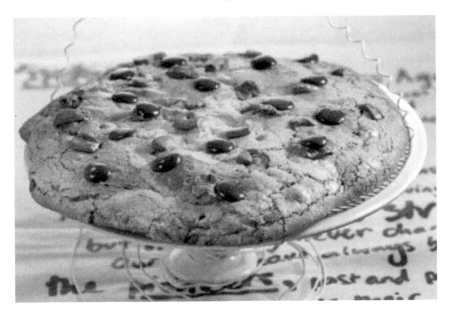

Ingredients:

- 2 tablespoons almond butter, softened
- 1/2 cup coconut sugar
- 1 egg white
- 2 teaspoon vanilla extract
- 2/3 cup almond flour
- 1 teaspoon bicarbonate of soda
- 1 cup sugar-free chocolate chips
- 1/4 cup sugar free chocolate, chopped (to garnish)

How to prepare:

1. Adjust the oven to 350 degrees F.

2. Combine cream with coconut sugar, and butter until smooth.
3. Whisk in egg white and vanilla. Add baking soda and flour.
4. Mix well until smooth then fold in chocolate chips.
5. Divide the batter into small flat cookies over a baking sheet.
6. Bake for 14 minutes.
7. Top the giant cookie with chocolate.
8. Serve.

Preparation time: 10 minutes
Cooking time: 15 minutes
Total time: 25 minutes
Servings: 4

Nutritional Values:

- *Calories 271*
- *Total Fat 4 g*
- *Saturated Fat 1 g*
- *Cholesterol 0 mg*
- *Sodium 263 mg*
- *Total Carbs 9.6 g*
- *Sugar 0.1 g*
- *Fiber 3.8 g*
- *Protein 7.6 g*

Cod Nuggets

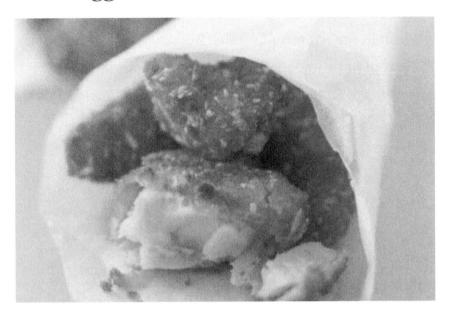

Ingredients:

- 2 cup vegetable oil, for deep-frying
- 2 cups skinless cod fillet, cut into chunks
- 1/2 cups almond flour
- salt
- pepper
- 2 medium egg whites, beaten
- 1 cup natural breadcrumbs
- 1/4 cup rolled oats

How to prepare:

1. Grind oats in a processor and then mix them with breadcrumbs.

2. Preheat oil in a saucepan.

3. Mix flour with seasonings and dip the cod in the flour mixture.

4. Now dip the chunks in the egg white whisk and then in breadcrumbs' mixture.

5. Deep fry them for 4 minutes until golden brown.

6. Serve.

Preparation time: 10 minutes

Cooking time: 05 minutes

Total time: 15 minutes

Servings: 4

Nutritional Values:

- *Calories 199*
- *Total Fat 7g*
- *Saturated Fat 3.5 g*
- *Cholesterol 125 mg*
- *Total Carbs 7.2 g*
- *Sugar 1.4 g*
- *Fiber 2.1 g*
- *Sodium 135 mg*
- *Protein 4.7 g*

Sesame Prawn Toast

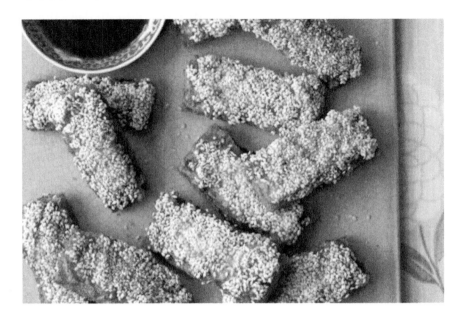

Ingredients:

For the prawn paste

- 4 1/4 cup raw prawns, peeled
- ½ x 8oz.inn water chestnuts, finely chopped
- 1/2 cups minced pork
- 1 egg white
- ½ bunch spring onions, white parts, finely chopped
- 1 tablespoon grated root ginger
- 2 teaspoon coconut aminos
- 2 teaspoon sugar
- 2 teaspoon sesame oil

For the toast

- 10 thin slices slightly stale white bread
- 3 tablespoon white sesame seeds
- 41/4 cup groundnut or vegetable oil

How to prepare:

1. Chop the prawns roughly and make mince from them.
2. Combine this mince with pork and other paste ingredients.
3. Remove crust from the bread and slice into 3 rectangles.
4. Spread the prawn mixture on each slice and top it with sesame seeds.
5. Heat oil in a wok and add toasts using a slotted spoon with the paste side down.
6. Deep fry them for 3 minutes. Turn carefully and fry for 2 minutes more.
7. Place them on a plat, layered with paper towel.
8. Serve.

Preparation time: 10 minutes

Cooking time: 10 minutes

Total time: 20 minutes

Servings: 4

Nutritional Values:

- *Calories 151*
- *Total Fat 3.4 g*
- *Saturated Fat 7 g*
- *Cholesterol 20 mg*
- *Total Carbs 6.4 g*
- *Sugar 2.1 g*
- *Fiber 4.8 g*
- *Sodium 136 mg*
- *Protein 4.2 g*

Cauliflower Popcorn

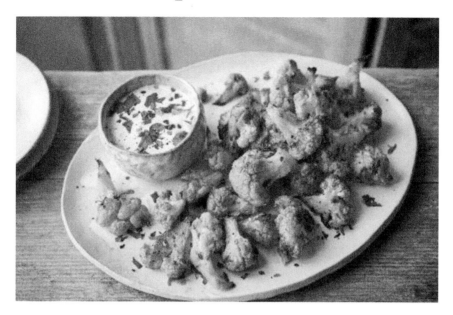

Ingredients:
- 1 large cauliflower, trimmed
- 1 teaspoon ground cumin
- 1 teaspoon ground turmeric
- 1 teaspoon crushed chili pepper flakes
- ½ teaspoon sea salt
- 2 tablespoon light olive oil

How to prepare:
1. Adjust the oven to 400 degrees F. Dice the cauliflower into small chunks.
2. Toss it with remaining ingredients and spread onto a baking sheet.
3. Bake for 30 minutes then serve.

Preparation time: 10 minutes

Cooking time: 30 minutes

Total time: 40 minutes

Servings: 4

Nutritional Values:

- *Calories 165*
- *Total Fat 3 g*
- *Saturated Fat 0.2 g*
- *Cholesterol 09 mg*
- *Sodium 7.1 mg*
- *Total Carbs 17.5 g*
- *Sugar 1.1 g*
- *Fiber 0.5 g*
- *Protein 2.2 g*

Sugar snap pea snacks

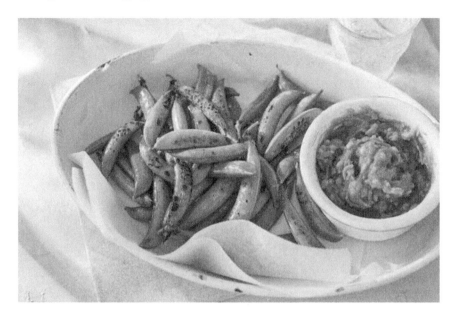

Ingredients:

- 1 tablespoon oil
- 2 cupssugar snapp peas
- 1 teaspoon sesame oil
- 1 teaspoon crushed chillies flakes
- For the satay dip
- 2/3 cup crunchy peanut butter
- 2 tablespoon coconut aminos
- 1 lime, zested and juiced
- 1 teaspoon coconut sugar
- 1 garlic clove, crushed
- 1 teaspoon ginger, grated

How to prepare:

1. Preheat the frying pan with ½ tablespoon oil. Saute peas for 5 minutes per side.
2. Transfer them to plat, lined with paper towel
3. Mix peanut butter with lime juice, sugar, garlic, coconut aminos, ginfger, and 4 tablesppons of water.
4. Toss in charred peas and serve with crushed chilies flakes and sesame oil on top.
5. Serve.

Preparation time: 5 minutes

Cooking time: 5 minutes

Total time: 10 minutes

Servings: 4

Nutritional Values:

- *Calories 102*
- *Total Fat 1 g*
- *Saturated Fat 0 g*
- *Cholesterol 0 mg*
- *Sodium 138 mg*
- *Total Carbs 24 g*
- *Fibre 0g*
- *Sugar 0 g*
- *Protein 2 g*

Flapjacks

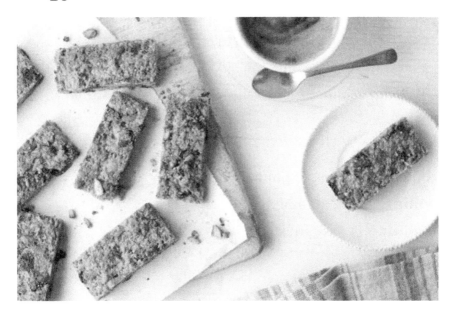

Ingredients:

- ¼ cup almond butter
- ¼ cup golden syrup
- ¼ cup coconut sugar
- 1 1/4 cup oats
- 1/4 cup sunflower seeds
- 1 teaspoon sesame seeds
- 1/3 cup dried apricot pieces, finely chopped
- 1/3 cup sultanas

How to prepare:

1. Adjust the oven to 320 degrees F. Layer a 20 cm baking pan with parchment paper.

2. Mix butter with sugar and golden syrup in a pan over medium heat.
3. Stir in all remaining ingredients.
4. Pour this mixture onto the baking pan and press it gently.
5. Bake for 20minutess the slice into 16 squares.
6. Serve.

Preparation time: 10 minutes
Cooking time: 20 minutes
Total time: 30 minutes
Servings: 6

Nutritional Values:

- *Calories 209*
- *Total Fat 0.5 g*
- *Saturated Fat 11.7 g*
- *Cholesterol 58 mg*
- *Sodium 163 mg*
- *Total Carbs 19.9 g*
- *Fiber 1.5 g*
- *Sugar 0.3 g*
- *Protein 3.3 g*

Crab cakes

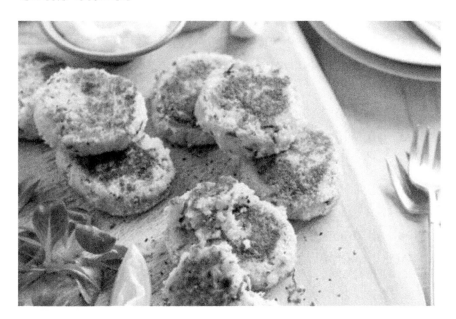

Ingredients:

- 2 cups (10oz) white crab meat
- 1 shallot, finely chopped
- small handful coriander leaves, finely chopped
- 2 limes, 1 zested and one cut into wedges
- 1/2 cups (3 1/2oz) white gluten-free bread
- 4 1/2 tablespoon mayonnaise, plus extra to serve
- pinch of sea salt
- pinch of black pepper
- 1 egg white, beaten
- sunflower oil, to fry

How to prepare:

1. Add bread to the processor and grind to form crumbs.

2. Mix crab meat with lime juice, shallot and coriander, and breadcrumb.
3. Adjust seasoning with pepper and salt. Divide the batter into 12 small balls and flatten them slightly with your hands.
4. Refrigerate for 20 minutes covered with plastic.
5. Beat egg white in a bowl and keep breadcrumbs in the other.
6. First dip that pancakes in the egg and then covers with crumbs.
7. Heat oil and sear the crab cakes for 3 minutes per side until golden brown.
8. Serve.

Preparation time: 10 minutes
Cooking time: 10 minutes
Total time: 20 minutes
Servings: 4

Nutritional Values:
- *Calories 237*
- *Total Fat 19.8 g*
- *Saturated Fat 1.4 g*
- *Cholesterol 10 mg*
- *Sodium 719 mg*
- *Total Carbs 55.1 g*
- *Fiber 0.9 g*
- *Sugar 1.4 g*
- *Protein 17.8 g*

Chapter 6: The 21-day blueprint for reducing acid damage, revving up metabolism, and staying healthy for life:

Days	Breackfast	Lunch	Snack	Dinner	Dessert
1.	Spiced Apricot Oats	Pepper and Onion Tart	Halloumi Fries	Seafood paella	Carrot Cupcakes
2.	Banana and blackberry smoothie bowl	Oat and Chickpea Dumplings	Mini pea pancakes	Sicilian Seafood Stew	Giant Chocolate Chip Cookie
3.	Banana breakfast loaf	Mushroom risotto	Cod Nuggets	Seafood Stew	Flapjacks

4.	Plum and almond porridge	Spaghetti with watercress and pea pesto	Sesame Prawn Toast	Fritto Misto with gremolata	Carrot Cupcakes
5.	Bircher muesli	Vegetarian pasta bakes with halloumi	Cauliflower Popcorn	Fish soup	Giant Chocolate Chip Cookie
6.	Banana and mango smoothie	Broccoli pesto penne with chili and garlic	Sugar snap pea snacks	Fritto Misto	Flapjacks

7.	Moroccan fritters	Veggie rice bowl	Crab cakes	Chicken Chasseur	Carrot Cupcakes
8.	Pancakes with avocado	Thai tofu and red cabbage bowl	Halloumi Fries	Smoky chicken traybake	Giant Chocolate Chip Cookie
9.	Dutch pancakes	Vegan shepherd's pie	Mini pea pancakes	Chicken and Orzo Bake	Flapjacks
10.	French crepes with bananas	Vegan vegetable curry	Cod Nuggets	One-Pot Roast	Carrot Cupcakes
11.	Spiced Apricot Oats	Pepper and Onion	Sesame Prawn Toast	Beef curry	Giant Chocolate

		Tart			Chip Cookie
12.	Banana and blackberry smoothie bowl	Oat and Chickpea Dumplings	Cauliflower Popcorn	Beef schnitzel	Flapjacks
13.	Banana breakfast loaf	Mushroom risotto	Sugar snap pea snacks	Beef Massaman Curry	Carrot Cupcakes
14.	Plum and almond porridge	Spaghetti with watercress and pea pesto	Crab cakes	Barbecued rump of beef in Dijon	Giant Chocolate Chip Cookie
15.	Bircher	Vegetari	Halloum	Roast rib of	Flapjac

	muesli	an pasta bakes with halloumi	i Fries	beef	ks
16.	Banana and mango smoothie	Broccoli pesto penne with chili and garlic	Mini pea pancakes	Beef Wellington with Stilton	Carrot Cupcakes
17.	Moroccan fritters	Veggie rice bowl	Cod Nuggets	Marinated lamb steaks	Giant Chocolate Chip Cookie
18.	Pancakes with avocado	Thai tofu and red	Sesame Prawn Toast	Lamb kofta curry	Flapjacks

		cabbage bowl		
19.	Dutch pancakes	Vegan shepherd's pie	Cauliflower Popcorn	Mediterranean Lamb Stew with Olives	Carrot Cupcakes
20.	French crepes with bananas	Vegan vegetable curry	Sugar snap pea snacks	Herb and spiced lamb	Giant Chocolate Chip Cookie
21.	Spiced Apricot Oats	Roast rib of beef	Crab cakes	Mushroom risotto	Flapjacks

Chapter-7. FDA's pH Food List:

Item	Approximate pH
Abalone	6.10 - 6.50
Abalone mushroom	5.00 -
Aloe Vera	6.10
Aloe Juice	6.00 - 6.80
Anchovies	6.50
Anchovies, stuffed w/capers, in olive oil	5.58
Antipasto	5.60 -
Apple, baked with sugar	3.20 - 3.55
Apple, eating	3.30 - 4.00
Apples	
Delicious	3.90
Golden Delicious	3.60
Jonathan	3.33
McIntosh	3.34
Juice	3.35 - 4.00
Sauce	3.10 - 3.60
Winesap	3.47
Apricots	3.30 - 4.80
Canned	3.40 - 3.78
Dried, stewed	3.30 - 3.51

Nectar	3.78
Pureed,	3.42 - 3.83
Strained	3.72 - 3.95
Arrowroot Crackers	6.63 - 6.80
Arrowroot Cruel	6.37 - 6.87
Artichokes	5.50 - 6.00
Artichokes, canned, acidified	4.30 - 4.60
Artichokes, French, cooked	5.60 - 6.00
Artichokes, Jerusalem, cooked	5.93 - 6.00
Asparagus	6.00 - 6.70
Buds	6.70
Stalks	6.10
Asparagus, cooked	6.03 - 6.16
Asparagus, canned	5.00 - 6.00
Asparagus, frozen, cooked	6.35 - 6.48
Asparagus, green, canned	5.20 - 5.32
Asparagus, strained	4.80 - 5.09
Avocados	6.27 - 6.58
Baby corn	5.20 -
Baby Food Soup, unstrained	5.95 - 6.05
Bamboo Shoots +	5.10 - 6.20
Bamboo Shoots, preserved	3.50 - 4.60
Bananas	4.50 - 5.20
Bananas, red	4.58 - 4.75

Banana, yellow	5.00 - 5.29
Barley, cooked	5.19 - 5.32
Basil pesto	4.90
Bass, sea, broiled	6.58 - 6.78
Bass, striped, broiled	6.50 - 6.70
Beans	5.60 - 6.50
Black	5.78 - 6.02
Boston style	5.05 - 5.42
Kidney	5.40 - 6.00
Lima	6.50
Soy	6.00 - 6.60
String	5.60
Wax	5.30 - 5.70
Beans, pork & tomato sauce, canned	5.10 - 5.80
Beans, refried	5.90
Beans, vegetarian, tomato sauce, canned	5.32
Beets	5.30 - 6.60
Beets, cooked	5.23 - 6.50
Beets, canned, acidified	4.30 - 4.60
Beets, canned	4.90 - 5.80
Beets, chopped	5.32 - 5.56
Beets, strained	5.32 - 5.56
Bird's nest soup	7.20 - 7.60

Blackberries, Washington	3.85 - 4.50
Blueberries, Maine	3.12 - 3.33
Blueberries, frozen	3.11 - 3.22
Bluefish, Boston, filet, broiled	6.09 - 6.50
Bran	
Flakes	5.45 - 5.67
All Bran	5.59 - 6.19
Bread, white	5.00 - 6.20
Bread, Boston, brown	6.53
Bread, Cracked wheat	5.43 - 5.50
Bread, pumpernickel	5.40 -
Bread, Rye	5.20 - 5.90
Bread, whole wheat	5.47 - 5.85
Breadfruit, cooked	5.33
Broccoli, cooked	6.30 - 6.52
Broccoli, frozen, cooked	6.30 - 6.85
Broccoli, canned	5.20 - 6.00
Brussels sprout	6.00 - 6.30
Buttermilk	4.41 - 4.83
Cabbage	5.20 - 6.80
Green	5.50 - 6.75
Red	5.60 - 6.00
Savoy	6.30
White	6.20

Cactus	4.70
Calamari (Squid)	5.80
Cantaloupe	6.13 - 6.58
Capers	6.00
Carp	6.00
Carrots	5.88 - 6.40
Carrots, canned	5.18 - 5.22
Carrots, chopped	5.30 - 5.56
Carrots, cooked	5.58 - 6.03
Carrots, pureed	4.55 - 5.80
Carrots, strained	5.10 - 5.10
Cauliflower	5.60
Cauliflower, cooked	6.45 - 6.80
Caviar, American	5.70 - 6.00
Celery	5.70 - 6.00
Celery, cooked	5.37 - 5.92
Celery Knob, cooked	5.71 - 5.85
Cereal, strained	6.44 - 6.45
Chayote (mirliton), cooked	6.00 - 6.30
Cheese, American, mild	4.98
Cheese, Camembert	7.44
Cheese, Cheddar	5.90
Cheese, Cottage	4.75 - 5.02
Cheese, Cream, Philadelphia	4.10 - 4.79
Cheese Dip	5.80

Cheese, Deem	5.40
Cheese, Old English	6.15
Cheese, Roquefort	5.10 - 5.98
Cheese, Parmesan	5.20 - 5.30
Cheese, Snippy	5.18 - 5.2l
Cheese, Stilton	5.70
Cheese, Swiss Gruyere	5.68 - 6.62
Cherries, California	4.01 - 4.54
Cherries, frozen	3.32 - 3.37
Cherries, black, canned	3.82 - 3.93
Cherries, Maraschino	3.47 - 3.52
Cherries, red, Water pack	3.25 - 3.82
Cherries, Royal Ann	3.80 - 3.83
Chicory	5.90 - 6.05
Chili Sauce, acidified	2.77 - 3.70
Chives	5.20 - 6.31
Clams	6.00 - 7.10
Clam Chowder, New England	6.40
Coconut, fresh	5.50 - 7.80
Coconut milk	6.10 - 7.00
Coconut preserves	3.80 - 7.00
Codfish, boiled	5.30 - 6.10
Cod Liver	6.20
Conch	7.52 - 8.40
Congee	6.40

Corn	5.90 - 7.30
Corn, canned	5.90 - 6.50
Corn Flakes	4.90 - 5.38
Corn, frozen, cooked	7.33 - 7.68
Corn, Golden Bantam, cooked on the cob	6.22 - 7.04
Crab Meat	6.50 - 7.00
Crabapple Jelly, corn	2.93 - 3.02
Cranberry Juice, canned	2.30 - 2.52
Crabmeat, cooked	6.62 - 6.98
Cream, 20 percent	6.50 - 6.68
Cream, 40 percent	6.44 - 6.80
Cream of Asparagus	6.10
Cream of Coconut, canned	5.51 - 5.87
Cream of Potato soup	6.00
Cream of Wheat, cooked	6.06 - 6.16
Chrysanthemum drink	6.50
Cucumbers	5.12 - 5.78
Cucumbers, Dill pickles	3.20 - 3.70
Cucumbers, pickled	4.20 - 4.60
Curry sauce	6.00
Curry Paste, acidified	4.60 - 4.80
Cuttlefish	6.30
Dates, canned	6.20 - 6.40
Dates, Dromedary	4.14 - 4.88

Dungeness Crab Meat	
Eggplant	5.50 - 6.50
Eggs, new-laid, whole	6.58
White	7.96
Yolk	6.10
Eel	6.20
Escarole	5.70 - 6.00
Enchilada sauce	4.40 - 4.70
Fennel (Anise)	5.48 - 5.88
Fennel, cooked	5.80 - 6.02
Figs, Calamyrna	5.05 - 5.98
Figs, canned	4.92 - 5.00
Flounder, boiled	6.10 - 6.90
Flounder, fi1et, broiled	6.39 - 6.89
Four bean salad	5.60
Fruit cocktail	3.60 - 4.00
Garlic	5.80
Gelatin Dessert	2.60
Gelatin, plain jell	6.08
Gherkin	
Ginger	5.60 - 5.90
Ginseng, Korean drink	6.00 - 6.50
Gooseberries	2.80 - 3.10
Graham Crackers	7.10 - 7.92
Grapes, canned	3.50 - 4.50

Grapes, Concord	2.80 - 3.00
Grapes, Lady Finger	3.51 - 3.58
Grapes, Malaga	3.71 - 3.78
Grapes, Niagara	2.80 - 3.27
Grapes, Ribier	3.70 - 3.80
Grapes, Seedless	2.90 - 3.82
Grapes, Tokyo	3.50 - 3.84
Grapefruit	3.00 - 3.75
Grapefruit, canned	3.08 - 3.32
Grapefruit Juice, canned	2.90 - 3.25
Grass jelly	5.80 - 7.20
Greens, Mixed, chopped	5.05 - 5.22
Greens, Mixed, strained	5.22 - 5.30
Grenadine Syrup	2.31
Guava nectar	5.50
Guava, canned	3.37 - 4. 10
Guava Jelly	3.73
Haddock, Filet, broiled	6.17 - 6.82
Hearts of Palm	5.70
Herring	6.10
Hominy, cooked	6.00 - 7.50
Honey	3.70 - 4.20
Honey Aloe	4.70
Horseradish, freshly ground	5.35
Huckleberries, cooked with	3.38 - 3.43

sugar	
Jackfruit	4.80 - 6.80
Jam, fruit	3.50 - 4.50
Jellies, fruit	3.00 - 3.50
Jujube fruit	5.20
Junket type Dessert:	
Raspberry	6.27
Vanilla	6.49
Kale, cooked	6.36 - 6.80
Ketchup	3.89 - 3.92
Kippered, Herring, Marshall	5.75 - 6.20
Herring, Pickled	4.50 - 5.00
Kelp	6.30
Kumquat, Florida	3.64 - 4.25
Leeks	5.50 - 6.17
Leeks, cooked	5.49 - 6.10
Lemon Juice	2.00 - 2.60
Lentils, cooked	6.30 - 6.83
Lentil Soup	5.80
Lettuce	5.80 - 6.15
Lettuce, Boston	5.89 - 6.05
Lettuce, Iceberg	5.70 - 6.13
Lime Juice	2.00 - 2.35
Lime	2.00 - 2.80
Lobster bisque	6.90 -

Lobster soup	5.70
Lobster, cooked	7.10 - 7.43
Loganberries	2.70 - 3.50
Lotus Root	6.90 -
Lychee	4.70 - 5.01
Macaroni, cooked	5.10 - 6.41
Mackerel, King, boiled	6.26 - 6.50
Mackerel, Spanish, broiled	6.07 - 6.36
Mackerel, canned	5.90 - 6.40
Mangoes, ripe	3.40 - 4.80
Mangoes, green	5.80 - 6.00
Mangosteen	4.50 -5.00
Maple syrup	5.15
Maple syrup, light (Acidified)	4.60
Matzos	5.70
Mayhaw (a variety of strawberry)	3.27 - 3.86
Melba Toast	5.08 - 5.30
Melon, Casaba	5.78 - 6.00
Melons, Honeydew	6.00 - 6.67
Melons, Persian	5.90 - 6.38
Milk, cow	6.40 - 6.80
Milk, Acidophilus	4.09 - 4.25
Milk, condensed	6.33
Milk evaporated	5.90 - 6.30

Milk, Goat's	6.48
Milk, peptonized	7.10
Milk, Sour, fine curd	4.70 - 5.65
Milkfish	5.30
Mint Jelly	3.01
Molasses	4.90 - 5.40
Muscadine (A variety of grape)	3.20 - 3.40
Mushrooms	6.00 - 6.70
Mushrooms, cooked	6.00 - 6.22
Mushroom Soup, Cream of, canned	5.95 - 6.40
Mussels	6.00 - 6.85
Mustard	3.55 - 6.00
Nata De Coco	5.00
Nectarines	3.92 - 4.18
Noodles, boiled	6.08 - 6.50
Oatmeal, cooked	6.20 - 6.60
Octopus	6.00 - 6.50
Okra, cooked	5.50 - 6.60
Olives, black	6.00 - 7.00
Olives, green, fermented	3.60 - 4.60
Olives, ripe	6.00 -7.50
Onions, pickled	3.70 - 4.60
Onions, red	5.30 - 5.80

Onion white	5.37 - 5.85
Onions, yellow	5.32 - 5.60
Oranges, Florida	3.69 - 4.34
Oranges, Florida "color added."	3.60 - 3.90
Orange Juice, California	3.30 - 4.19
Orange, Juice Florida	3.30 - 4.15
Orange, Marmalade	3.00 - 3.33
Oysters	5.68 - 6.17
Oyster, smoked	6.00
Oyster mushrooms	5.00 - 6.00
Palm, the heart of	6.70
Papaya	5.20 - 6.00
Papaya Marmalade	3.53 - 4.00
Parsley	5.70 - 6.00
Parsnip	5.30 - 5.70
Parsnips, cooked	5.45 - 5.65
Pate	5.90
Peaches	3.30 - 4.05
Peaches, canned	3.70 - 4.20
Peaches, cooked with sugar	3.55 - 3.72
Peaches, frozen	3.28 - 3.35
Peanut Butter	6.28
Peanut Soup	7.5
Pears, Bartlett	3.50 - 4.60

Pears, canned	4.00 - 4.07
Pears, Sickle cooked w/sugar	4.04 - 4.21
Pear Nectar	4.03
Peas, canned	5.70 - 6.00
Peas, Chick, Garbanzo	6.48 - 6.80
Peas, cooked	6.22 - 6.88
Peas, dried (split green), cooked	6.45 - 6.80
Peas, dried (split yellow), cooked	6.43 - 6.62
Peas, frozen, cooked	6.40 - 6.70
Peas, pureed	4.90 - 5.85
Pea Soup, Cream of, Canned	5.70
Peas, strained	5.91 - 6.12
Peppers	4.65 - 5.45
Peppers, green	5.20 - 5.93
Persimmons	4.42 - 4.70
Pickles, fresh pack	5.10 - 5.40
Pimiento	4.40 - 4.90
Pimento, canned, acidified	4.40 - 4.60
Pineapple	3.20 - 4.00
Pineapple, canned	3.35 - 4.10
Pineapple Juice, canned	3.30 - 3.60
Plum Nectar	3.45
Plums, Blue	2.80 - 3.40

Plums, Damson	2.90 - 3.10
Plums, Frozen	3.22 - 3.42
Plums, Green Gage	3.60 - 4.30
Plums, Green Gage, canned	3.22 - 3.32
Plums, Red	3.60 - 4.30
Plums, spiced	3.64
Plums, Yellow	3.90 - 4.45
Pollack, filet, broiled	6.72 - 6.82
Pomegranate	2.93 - 3.20
Porgy, broiled	6.40 - 6.49
Pork & Beans, rts.	5.70
Potatoes	5.40 - 5.90
Mashed	5.10
Prunes, dried, stewed	3.63 - 3.92
Sweet	5.30 - 5.60
Tubers	5.70
Potato Soup	5.90
Prune Juice	3.95 - 3.97
Prune, pureed	3.60 - 4.30
Prune, strained	3.58 - 3.83
Puffed Rice	6.27 - 6.40
Puffed Wheat	5.26 - 5.77
Pumpkin	4.90 - 5.50
Quince, fresh, stewed	3.12 - 3.40
Quince Jelly	3.70

Radishes, red	5.85 - 6.05
Radishes, white	5.52 - 5.69
Raisins, seedless	3.80 - 4.10
Rambutan (Thailand)	4.90
Raspberries	3.22 - 3.95
Raspberries, frozen	3.18 - 3.26
Raspberries, New Jersey	3.50 - 3.82
Raspberry Jam	2.87 - 3.17
Razor Clams	6.20
Razor shell (sea asparagus)	6.00
Rattan, Thailand	5.20 -
Red Ginseng	5.50
Red Pepper Relish	3.10 - 3.62
Rhubarb, California, stewed	3.20 - 3.34
Rhubarb	3.10 - 3.40
Canned	3.40
Rice (all cooked)	
Brown	6.20 - 6.80
Krispies	5.40 - 5.73
White	6.00 - 6.70
Wild	6.00 - 6.50
Rolls, white	5.46 - 5.52
Romaine	5.78 - 6.06
Salmon, fresh, boiled	5.85 - 6.50
Salmon, fresh, broiled	5.36 - 6.40

Salmon, Red Alaska, canned	6.07 - 6.16
Salsa	
Sardines	5.70 - 6.60
Sardine, Portuguese, in olive oil	5.42 - 5.93
Satay sauce	5.00
Sauce, Enchilada	5.50 -
Sauce, Fish	4.93 - 5.02
Sauce, Shrimp	7.01 - 7.27
Sauerkraut	3.30 - 3.60
Scallion	6.20 -
Scallop	6.00
Scotch Broth.	5.92
Sea Snail (Top shell)	6.00
Shad Roe, sauteed	5.70 - 5.90
Shallots, cooked	5.30 - 5.70
Sherbet, raspberry	3.69
Sherry-wine	3.37
Shredded Ralston	5.32 - 5.60
Shredded Wheat	6.05 - 6.49
Shrimp	6.50 - 7.00

Shrimp Paste	5.00 - 6.77
Smelts, Sauteed	6.67 - 6.90
Soda Crackers	5.65 - 7.32
Soup	
Broccoli Cheese Soup, condensed	5.60 -
Chicken Broth, rts.	5.80
Corn Soup, condensed	6.80
Cream of Celery Soup, condensed	6.20 -
Cream of Mushroom, condensed	6.00 - 6.20
Cream style corn, condensed	5.70 - 5.80
Cream of Potato soup, condensed	5.80 -
Cream of shrimp soup, condensed	5.80
Minestrone condensed	5.40
New England Clam Chowder, condensed	6.00-
Oyster Stew, condensed	6.30 -

Tomato Rice Soup, condensed	5.50 -
Soy infant formula	6.60 - 7.00
Coconut aminos	4.40 - 5.40
Soybean curd (tofu)	7.20
Soybean milk	7.00
Spaghetti, cooked	5.97 - 6.40
Spinach	5.50 - 6.80
Spinach, chopped	5.38 - 5.52
Spinach, cooked	6.60 - 7.18
Spinach, frozen, cooked	6.30 - 6.52
Spinach, pureed	5.50 - 6.22
Spinach, strained	5.63 - 5.79
Squash, acorn, cooked	5.18 - 6.49
Squash, Kubbard, cooked	6.00 - 6.20
Squash, white, cooked	5.52 - 5.80
Squash, yellow, cooked	5.79 - 6.00
Squid	6.00 - 6.50
Sturgeon	6.20
Strawberries	3.00 - 3.90
Strawberries, California	3.32 - 3.50
Strawberries, frozen	3.21 - 3.32
Strawberry Jam	3.00 - 3.40
Straw mushroom	4.90

Sweet Potatoes	5.30 - 5.60
Swiss Chard, cooked	6.17 - 6.78
Tamarind	3.00 -
Tangerine	3.32 - 4.48
Taro syrup	4.50
Tea	7.20
Three-Bean Salad	5.40
Tofu (soybean Curd)	7.20
Tomatillo (resembling Cherry tomatoes)	3.83
Tomatoes	4.30 - 4.90
Tomatoes, canned	3.50 - 4.70
Tomatoes, Juice	4.10 - 4.60
Tomatoes, Paste	3.50 - 4.70
Tomatoes, Puree	4.30 - 4.47
Tomatoes, Strained	4.32 - 4.58
Tomatoes, Wine ripened	4.42 - 4.65
Tomato Soup, Cream of, canned	4.62
Trout, Sea, sauteed	6.20 - 6.33
Truffle	5.30 - 6.50
Tuna Fish, canned	5.90 - 6.20
Turnips	5.29 - 5.90
Turnip, greens, cooked	5.40 - 6.20
Turnip, white, cooked	5.76 - 5.85

Turnip, yellow, cooked	5.57 - 5.82
Vegetable Juice	3.90 - 4.30
Vegetable soup, canned	5.16
Vegetable soup, chopped	4.98 - 5.02
Vegetable soup, strained	4.99 - 5.00
Vermicelli, cooked	5.80 - 6.50
Vinegar	2.40 - 3.40
Vinegar, cider	3.10
Walnuts, English	5.42
Wax gourd drink	7.20
Water Chestnut	6.00 - 6.20
Watercress	5.88 - 6.18
Watermelon	5.18 - 5.60
Wheat Krispice	4.99 - 5.62
Wheaten	5.85 - 6.08
Wheaties	5.00 - 5.12
Worcestershire sauce	3.63 - 4.00
Yams, cooked	5.50 - 6.81
Yeast	5.65
Zucchini, cooked	5.69 - 6.10

Conclusion

In sum, the causes of acid reflux are diverse, so there is a firm demand for both treatments and preventative measures to alleviate the worsening of this health condition. More often than usual, our negative dietary habits and sleeplessness which trap us into the acid reflux cycle. Regardless of the cause, this dietary plan and a detailed account of the GERD can help everyone to fight the problem at hand while managing small and gradual changes in eating practices. With such a change in mindset, you can accomplish anything and push back the burning issue of acid reflux once and for all!

Printed in Great Britain
by Amazon

32578123R00098